# The Complete Guide to Joseph H. Pilates' Techniques of Physical Conditioning

## Praise for the First Edition

Recommended by:

- *Physical* magazine
- About.com, Physical Therapy Guide
- The Pilates Center of Austin
- Center of Balance (Mountain View, CA)
- The Pacific Northwest Inlander
- The Bodyworker.com

"This book offers a thorough, in-depth guide to Pilates exercises."

—*Pilates Insight.com*

"This is a very comprehensive book. It covers around 200 Pilates exercises. The introductory chapters are inspiring especially for anyone who experiences pain. Allen Menezes, the author, experienced a great deal of pain himself and seems to truly understand how to help people work with and through their pain....The introduction helps with an understanding of the method behind the movements and the concluding chapters actually offer some information that is a must...."

—*Pilates Fitness Journal,* August 2003

"A more in-depth book on Pilates that will appeal to teachers, some excellent information."

—*Bodyline LA*

"An excellent book that presents a wide variety of Pilates-based exercises, incorporating photographs with step-by-step instructions, key points, cautions, and variations. Nicely illustrated with good photography."

—Judd Robbins, Director of Central Internet Resource for Pilates' Instructors, Studios and Students (www.bodymind.net)

## What Readers Say

"Allan's Body Control Pilates Technique is the surest way I know to get back into shape fast. It gives maximum effect with minimum effort, and helps iron out the stresses life inflicts on the back. It addresses muscles you didn't even know existed that help to keep the body toned and fortified."

—Greta Scacchi, actress
(*The Red Violin, Emma, Presumed Innocent*)

"Have you tried every exercise program on the market only to quit after the first few lessons? That has been my experience until two weeks ago when I began a Pilates course. The instructor uses *The Complete Guide to the Pilates Method* as her instruction manual....With this book as a reference guide, I can continue the Pilates exercises at home and have quit being a quitter."

—Valerie, Perth, Australia

"Simply a great all-around book! I have had back trouble for about 15 years and within only 3 weeks of following the teachings of J.H. Pilates I have noticed considerable improvement in mobility, flexibility, and strength. The book has lots of valuable information over and above the clear description and illustration of exercises contained within and makes for very interesting reading even when taking it easy!"

—Graeme, Queensland, Australia

"I tried Pilates about 1 year ago and absolutely loved it! I used [this] book which provides lots of great details and background information essential to getting started."

—*Healthy Living* Editor @ Hippodamia

## TO MY WIFE, SONJA

*Project Credits*

Cover Design: Jinni Fontana Graphic Design
Photography: KC
Models: Simon Wood, Vanessa Wood, Allan Menezes, Nadine Jenkins, and Jennifer Scott
Illustrations: Daniel Matthieu
Book Design and Production: Jinni Fontana Graphic Design
Copy Editor: Kelley Blewster
Proofreader: Lee Rappold
Acquisitions Editor: Jeanne Brondino
Editor: Alexandra Mummery
Publicist: Lisa E. Lee
Foreign Rights Assistant: Elisabeth Wohofsky
Customer Service Manager: Christina Sverdrup
Order Fulfillment: Washul Lakdhon
Administrator: Theresa Nelson
Computer Support: Peter Eichelberger
Publisher: Kiran S. Rana

*Ordering*

Trade bookstores in the U.S. and Canada please contact:

Publishers Group West
1700 Fourth Street, Berkeley CA 94710
Phone: (800) 788-3123    Fax: (510) 528-3444

Hunter House books are available at bulk discounts for textbook course adoptions;
to qualifying community, health-care, and government organizations; and for special
promotions and fund-raising. For details please contact:

Special Sales Department
Hunter House Inc., PO Box 2914, Alameda CA 94501-0914
Phone: (510) 865-5282    Fax: (510) 865-4295
E-mail: sales@hunterhouse.com

Individuals can order our books from most bookstores, by calling
(800) 266-5592, or from our website at **www.hunterhouse.com**

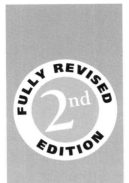

# THE COMPLETE GUIDE TO JOSEPH H. PILATES' TECHNIQUES OF PHYSICAL CONDITIONING

## With Special Help for Back Pain and Sports Training

### ALLAN MENEZES

*Founder of the Pilates Institute of Australasia and the Body Control Pilates Studios*

Physical fitness is the first

prerequisite of happiness.

— J. PILATES (1880–1967)

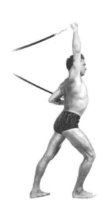

FULLY REVISED 2nd EDITION

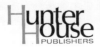
Hunter House
PUBLISHERS

Hunter House Inc., Publishers
PO Box 2914
Alameda CA 94501-0914

First published in Australia in 1998 by the Pilates Institute of Australasia Pty Ltd., P.O. Box 1046, North Sydney 2059, New South Wales, Australia. www.pilates.net.

Contrology®, Reformer®, and B-Line® are all Registered Trademarks in Australia and are used with permission by the Pilates Institute of Australasia.

Body Control Pilates™, Stable Spine™, and the Menezes Technique™ are Trademarks used by the Pilates Institute of Australasia P/L and Body Control Australia P/L.

The Pilates Institute of Australasia and Body Control Pilates are not associated with any organizations of the same or similar name outside Australia. Beware of imitations.

*Library of Congress Cataloging-in-Publication Data*

Menezes, Allan.
    The complete guide to Joseph H. Pilates' techniques of physical conditioning : with special help for back pain and sports training / by Allan Menezes.—2nd ed.
        p. cm.
    Includes bibliographical references.
    ISBN 0-89793-438-5 (pbk.)
1. Pilates method. I. Title: Joseph H. Pilates' techniques of physical conditioning. II. Title: Techniques of physical conditioning. III. Title.
RA781.M4 2004
613.7'1—dc22                                                    2004001431

Printed and Bound by Bang Printing, Brainerd, Minnesota

Manufactured in the United States of America

9 8 7 6 5 4 3 2 1          Second Edition          04 05 06 07 08

# CONTENTS

## 1
## WHY OUR BODIES NEED A REGULAR FITNESS PROGRAM

## 2
## MENTAL CONTROL OVER PHYSICAL MOVEMENT

## 3
## THE IMPORTANCE OF POSTURE

## 4
## MAKING YOUR PILATES WORKOUT EFFECTIVE AND SAFE

# 5
## THE WARM-UP

# 6
## THE ROUTINE FOR LOWER-BACK PAIN AND WEAK ABDOMINALS

# 7
## THE BASIC ROUTINE

# 8
## THE INTERMEDIATE ROUTINE

## 9

# The Advanced Routine

## 10

# More Challenging Exercises

## 11

# Theraband Routines

## 12

## MOVE YOURSELF OUT OF PAIN

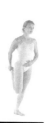

# About the Author

Allan Menezes is the founder and owner of Body Control Australia and the Body Control Pilates Studios, and the founder of the Pilates Institute of Australasia.

While in college, Allan suffered a debilitating back injury in a rugby accident, which hospitalized him and virtually ended his athletic career. After two years of chronic lower-back pain, he attended a Pilates studio in London in 1982. Six weeks of daily visits to the studio cured his back problem. This convinced him that a huge, untapped market—people with back pain—existed for the application of the Pilates method, and he changed careers to become an instructor with the Alan Herdman Studios. Allan introduced Pilates to Australia in November 1986, and he now runs two Body Control Pilates Studios in Sydney. He also conducts international teacher-training courses in AUSSIEpilates Method and manufactures equipment and produces videos and DVDs through the Pilates Institute of Australasia.

Allan has a lengthy history of participation in sports including tennis, swimming, squash, volleyball, basketball, cricket, track and field (where he set many records), karate, rugby, American football, cross-country running, skiing, and weight training. At the university level he was captain of his volleyball, basketball, and rugby teams. Throughout his sports career he sustained his fair share of injuries.

Allan received his Pilates Teacher Trainer Certification from the former Institute for the Pilates Method in Santa Fe, New Mexico, in 1992. He is also a former member of that organization's advisory board. In 1996 he founded the Pilates Institute of Australasia to ensure that consistently high standards in Pilates training were established. The institute's courses and workshops are accredited by the Australian Fitness Accreditation Council (AFAC).

Allan has lectured internationally on Joseph H. Pilates' unique techniques of body control, and he conducts workshops for the general public as well as for physiotherapists, medical practitioners, and other rehabilitation specialists.

The Body Control Pilates Studios and the Pilates Institute of Australasia have been featured in many of Australia's major magazines and newspapers. Allan has also been interviewed several times on television and radio, and was featured in *Entrepreneur International Magazine.*

Allan lives in Sydney with his wife, Sonja, and their daughters, Jessica, Analiese, and Monique.

# FOREWORD

This new edition is even better than the last. It is designed for everyone in search of a leaner, stronger, more flexible body. It is certainly geared to providing you with what we are all searching for from any exercise program: results!

This book still contains the most comprehensive and detailed instruction on Pilates exercises available anywhere in the world. The combination of precise detail and helpful illustrations provides a clear and easy-to-understand resource for both the novice and the Pilates professional. Those who can benefit from this book range from triathletes to ballet dancers, from new mothers to those who suffer from lower-back pain.

I found the section on the B-Line of great assistance in applying abdominal bracing in a different, effective style. Allan has now gone a step further: his introduction of the concept of the B-Line-Core has once again set the standard for others to follow. Applying it to every physical movement, whether a person is exercising or not, will afford extra bodily support for everyday activities not found in other exercise programs.

This book is more than an inspiration to those who have attempted other exercise programs and found them wanting. It will take you farther, even if you are currently using Pilates as part of your fitness program. By following this guide you will both discover and learn to understand your body. The techniques described here will deliver an energized body that also looks good!

Allan has contributed tremendously to the emergence of Pilates worldwide. He is certainly one of its foremost practitioners. He doesn't sit still—he is continuously developing and expanding his style and his thinking for the benefit of the reader and of Pilates instructors everywhere. The fact that this book is used as an instructor's manual worldwide further confirms his position as a Master Pilates Practitioner. Allan's willingness to share his insights is to be congratulated.

Make the most of this book—it delivers results!

*— Peter Green, D.O.*
*Course Coordinator of Osteopathy*
*University of Western Sydney*
*Sydney, Australia*

This book is an improved version of my previous book, which I wrote to answer the need for an up-to-date version of the exercise routine developed by Joseph Pilates in the early 1920s. It is a well-accepted fact that Joe Pilates was fifty years ahead of his time. Even Pilates himself believed that to be true. Many who respect and honor his work feel that if Joe were alive today, he would have taken much of his work to the next level. This book attempts to do that.

Pilates' outstanding insights into the movement of the human body came naturally to him. Many advanced Pilates instructors throughout the world, who have been followers of the method for many years, have developed those same insights. By utilizing Joe's techniques, they have developed variations that in many cases are improvements on the original movements. As much as possible, I have presented here both the original versions of the movements and variations that have been developed over time, including routines that cater to those with lower-back pain.

This book really began when I first discovered Joseph Pilates' techniques in London in 1982. Two years previously, while in college studying for a business degree, I had injured my back in a rugby game. After several months in London, I began attending the Alan Herdman Studios, where I learned some of the best grounding in Pilates I have ever encountered. Alan is one of the master teachers of the method.

My rugby injury was so severe that I lay in a hospital bed for ten days and was allowed only liquids for nourishment. The diagnosis at the time was a slipped disc. X rays showed no abnormalities, and no scans were taken. For the following two years I visited almost every practitioner I could find in the hope of alleviating my pain.

Then, in London, my father handed me an introductory voucher for a "new" method that was being taught in a small basement studio. Little did I know that the method was then almost sixty years new. After I attended Pilates classes every day for six weeks, my back pain disappeared! Regular sessions followed for the next two or three years, and my back pain has not returned to this day, even though I run and play squash. (Years later I discovered from a CAT scan that I had actually herniated my discs at the fourth and fifth lumbar vertebrae.)

I was an instant convert to the Pilates method. The one drawback was that my original instructors had very little anatomical or athletic knowledge. They could not explain the whys and wherefores of a particular movement or its application to me as an ex-athlete.

My next step was to devise my own Pilates-based routines for improving my performance in squash, volleyball, and other sports. I also developed programs for other fitness enthusiasts. My variations required more exertion and were more challenging because they targeted specific muscle groups. They proved to be popular.

It was in 1986 that I established the first Pilates studio in the southern hemisphere with the Body Control Pilates Studios in Sydney. *(There is no connection with any other studio that has the same or a similar name outside of Australia and New Zealand.)* In 1994, after setting up two more studios, I established the first true franchise of a Pilates-based instruction studio. Two years later I founded the Pilates Institute of Australasia to cater to the growing demand for quality training and to provide accredited workshops and courses in Pilates.

Over the years I have created rules and formulas that have helped my staff and other teachers around the world to gain better results for their clients. I have named this new style AUSSIE*pilates*. Parts of it are included in this book. A more comprehensive book on AUSSIE*pilates* will be available in late 2004. Some of the major differences between the traditional Pilates method and AUSSIE*pilates* include the method of breathing (described in the sections on breathing in Chapters 2 and 3), the introduction of the Stamina Stretch (Exercise 2-2), and the description of the Stable Spine (Chapter 3).

As the demand for Pilates continues to grow, this will be an invaluable text for those wishing to reduce their niggling aches and pains. The book will also be an important resource for those wishing to become familiar with the basic steps involved in sensible body maintenance and for those embarking on a career in the growing Pilates industry. The techniques presented here offer a basis not only for perfection in movement but also for physical rehabilitation. I hope that you will learn and benefit from the ideas outlined in this book for a better body, a healthier mind, and limitless energy.

## ACKNOWLEDGEMENTS

*My thanks go to all my associates, who have been extremely patient during the development of this book. I thank them for the input they have provided and for their help in expanding the Body Control Pilates Studios (Australasia). Thanks to my father for handing me the voucher that changed my life and started an industry in Australia. To my mother, who without my knowing it at the time gave me my best motivation. To my clients, past and present, who have all contributed to the refinement of the routines by allowing me over the years to test new exercises and perfect old ones. Most important, my thanks and appreciation go to my wife, Sonja, who has displayed the ultimate in patience and encouragement through many frustrating moments in this book's long journey, and who has contributed enormously, on both the practical and emotional level, to the expansion of the organization. What a source of determination, perseverance, and inspiration she is to both me and the children.*

*I also wish to thank Vanessa Wood, Simon Wood, Jennifer Scott, and Nadine Jenkins for modeling for the photos.*

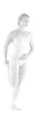

## WHO WAS JOSEPH PILATES
## AND WHAT IS THE PILATES METHOD?

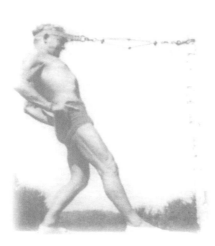

Joseph Humbertus Pilates was born in 1880 near Düsseldorf, Germany. He grew up suffering from rickets, asthma, and rheumatic fever. Like so many individuals inflicted with potentially devastating chronic illnesses who have gone on to excel in the area of physical achievement and innovation, Pilates became obsessed with the frailties of the body and was determined to overcome his own afflictions. As a teenager, he became skilled in gymnastics, skiing, and skin diving. He studied the musculature of the human body. Armed with a determination to work his body into a state of better health, by age fourteen he had improved his physical condition enough so that he was posing for anatomical drawings. His studies also included Eastern forms of exercise. When he merged these with his Western studies of physiology and movement, what has become known as the Pilates method was born. Pilates named his method Contrology.

In 1912 Joe went to England, where he became a boxer, circus performer, and self-defense instructor. When World War I erupted he and other German nationals were incarcerated in Lancaster and on the Isle of Man as enemy aliens. Many of his fellow internees, by following his exercise regime, emerged unscathed from an influenza epidemic that swept the nation, killing thousands. Others in the camp who were disabled by wartime diseases also benefited from Joe's innovative approach to physical fitness. He devised a forerunner of modern exercise equipment by removing the bedsprings from beneath the beds and attaching them to the walls above the patients' beds, allowing them to exercise while lying down. This permitted the patients to remain stable despite their injuries, while at the same time mobilizing themselves, strengthening their muscles, and emerging fitter and healthier than they would have if they had remained immobile during their convalescence.

When World War I ended, Joe Pilates returned to Germany, where he continued to develop his work. In 1926, he felt his ideals did not match those of the new German army, and he decided to emigrate to the United States. On the journey across the Atlantic, he met Clara, a nurse, who became his wife. "We talked so much about health and the need to keep the body healthy, we decided to open a physical fitness studio," said Clara. This was when the dance world became exposed to Pilates' teachings. Rudolf von Laban, the founder of Labanotation, incorporated several of Joe's principles into his teaching, as did Hanya Holm, Martha Graham, George Balanchine, and other choreographers.

From the start, Pilates was embraced by the dance world with great fervor. Consequently, more than 80 percent of Pilates-based teachers around the world come from a dance background. The movements, fluid in nature and designed to lengthen the muscles, have a balletic appearance to them. To apply the Pilates method to a tennis player, rugby fullback, or baseball pitcher, however, would be extremely difficult unless the instructor has played that sport or otherwise has a strong knowledge of athletic movement. This is because dance, unlike these sports, generally places equal physical demand on both sides of the body. For this reason, a dance-based instructor should ideally be trained in these other disciplines before practicing Pilates with athletes.

Because the Pilates method has expanded to areas outside the dance world, I have structured this book so that it can be used by anyone who wishes to learn the movements of the method, from basic to advanced. It is meant to be a definitive guide for those wishing to follow a sensible exercise program that produces results.

## THE BENEFITS OF REGULAR, PILATES-BASED EXERCISE

How does participating in regular exercise benefit us? Consider the following two opinions. Joseph Pilates in 1945 defined fitness as "the attainment and maintenance of a uniformly devel-oped body with a sound mind fully capable of naturally, easily, and satisfactorily performing our many and varied daily tasks with spontaneous zest and pleasure."

A recent report by the surgeon general of the United States, after decades of research on the effects of physical activity and health, reported that regular physical activity provides the following benefits:

- It reduces the risk of dying prematurely.
- It reduces the risk of dying from heart disease.
- It reduces the risk of developing diabetes.
- It reduces the risk of developing high blood pressure.
- It helps reduce blood pressure in people who already have high blood pressure.
- It reduces the risk of developing colon cancer.
- It reduces feelings of depression and anxiety.
- It aids in controlling weight.
- It helps the aged become stronger and more mobile.
- It improves psychological well-being.

Based on these proven benefits the surgeon general's office formerly recommended that all Americans exercise for forty minutes three times per week. The guidelines were updated in 2003 to recommend that Americans exercise for one hour per day, *every* day! This increase is a reflection of the growing rate of obesity in the Western world, the increasing lack of physical activity, the decline in the quality of most Westerners' nutritional intake, and the rise in pollution levels in our environment, whether from secondhand smoke, car fumes, or other toxins.

But what sort of exercise program works best? Gyms, with their fast-circuit classes and weight machines, tend to encourage work on the muscle groups that are already strong. Consequently, the strong muscle groups remain strong (and can get bulkier) and the weaker ones remain weak, or become marginally stronger at best. In addition, with a gym routine, once a person stops following the regimen, the results disappear rather quickly. With Pilates exercises, by contrast, results may not happen immediately, but in the long run, the benefits are clear. In addition, when you stop practicing the method for a time, the results still stay with you. And if you restart, even after a two-year break, you will feel as if you had stopped only yesterday.

Furthermore, unlike the usual gym routines, which work the muscles from the outside of the body toward the inside, Pilates works from muscles deeper within the body toward the outside muscle groups. By working from the inside out, you develop a greater understanding of the body. Smaller muscle groups come into use, and you begin to discover muscles you never knew you had—or you may realize that what you once thought was fat actually hides a muscle! Finally, the method helps you to develop a control that is useful for performing a range of movements—from the simplest, such as walking up a flight of stairs, to the most complex, such as lifting an awkward load from a difficult position—without straining the back, shoulders, or other muscles.

In summary, the Pilates method aims to produce the following:

1. Fluidity and awareness of movement.

2. Mental focus and control over bodily movements without the need to concentrate on them.

3. A body that "thinks" for itself.

4. A healthy body both inside and out.

Pilates held a firm belief that he was fifty years ahead of his time. Even today, although the original method has changed as it has spread across the globe, the basic principles that form the foundation of the method still hold true. The principles have been refined over the years to incorporate a more in-depth explanation of the muscles being used and the benefits of each exercise. However, even the simplest of the routines can gently lead you to greater physical challenges, improved mental focus, and increased health benefits.

*Notes*

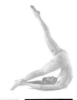

# Why Our Bodies Need a Regular Fitness Program

Man should

bear in mind

and ponder over

the Greek

admonition—

not too much,

not too little.

— J. Pilates

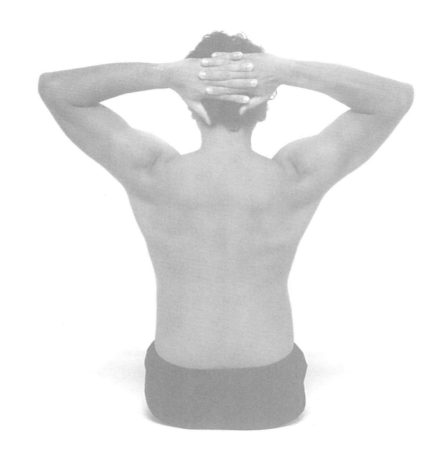

## THE EFFECTS OF LIFESTYLE AND STRESS ON THE BODY

Have you ever wished for more mental and physical stamina to aid you in playing longer with the children or grandchildren, completing the daily household chores, or even playing that extra game of tennis without becoming overfatigued? Have you ever wished to have more energy at the end of each day, rather than feeling drained? Have you ever wondered why so many people accept the back pain with which they live?

Why do we act and move the way we do? Why do we sometimes feel the same aches and pains as our parents did? Why do we develop new ones that our parents did not have? Will we acquire the same maladies that afflict the elderly people we know?

To a great extent, the answer to many such questions can be found in our current lifestyle: the fast pace of modern life, our eating habits, the effects of the greenhouse gases, and so on. Over many years, such a lifestyle can lead to mental and physical stress, which in turn causes the body to break down. This breakdown can manifest itself in several forms, ranging from mild allergies to severe and chronic aches and pains, to various types of injuries, or even to the breakdown of our personal relationships.

Such stresses can have a lasting effect on our lives. That is why we feel the urge to "get away from it all"—to escape to the mountains or the coast, to a quieter, more tranquil environment where we can "be ourselves." But at the end of our getaway we have to face it all over again. How are we supposed to cope with the pressures of life? How do we control our bodies so that they do not give way on us? Ultimately, how do we live longer, happier, healthier lives?

We can usually do very little about our inherited conditions. We cannot change the color of our eyes or the tone of our skin. And other, noninherited factors affect us as well. As we develop, we learn from those around us—our parents, our teachers, our peers, and others with whom we come in contact. Whether these experiences are good or bad, we tend to use them as reference points in our lives. We develop a mindset about what our abilities and capabilities are, formed in part by what we are told we can and cannot do.

We are affected by the choices we make in these formative years. Consider how as schoolchildren, many of us carried a heavy bag full of books, usually slinging it over one shoulder. One possible effect of this behavior is the development of scoliosis of the spine, a condition that can lead to back pain later in life if left untreated and if the contributing behavior continues throughout our developmental years.

As adults, we attempt to achieve more and to improve ourselves, usually by working long hours. As we try to accomplish higher goals, whether in the workplace or in our personal relationships, our physical and mental selves bear the brunt of our efforts at self-improvement. In order to handle difficult situations on a day-to-day basis and to sustain the changes we undertake, we require our bodies to provide us with increased mental and physical support and energy. The adage of "healthy body, healthy mind" is as true today as it has ever been. Even truer still is one of Joe Pilates' favorite quotes, from the German philosopher Frederich von Schiller: "It is the mind which controls the body." It is certainly of more benefit to be in control of your body rather than at its mercy!

## HOW WE ESTABLISH FAULTY PATTERNS OF MOVEMENT

Our workplace environment has become more sedentary, and our leisure time has followed suit. Children now spend more time in front of television and computer than ever before. These habits tend to follow them into adulthood. The era of the "couch potato" is upon us, and we have failed to notice that fact until almost too late. In addition, when our forebears began to walk upright many millennia ago, the resulting changes in how we moved our bodies led to a restriction of movements in our joints and an unbalanced configuration in our bodies and muscles.

This means that we tend to favor one group of muscles more than the others when we perform most of our day-to-day activities. For example,

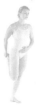

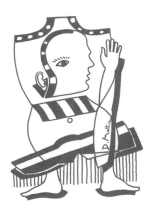

*Figure 1.*
*The unbalanced body*

each time we throw or kick a ball we tend to use the same arm or leg, women tend to hold a baby predominantly on the same hip, and we tend to hold a telephone to the same ear with the same hunched shoulder. These one-sided actions cause imbalances in the body. Even the way we walk, perhaps with an unnoticeably longer stride in one leg, can unbalance our musculoskeletal structures and can lead to back pain and even migraines.

Over time these continuous, repetitive movements become set in the memory of the muscle. These set movements, or *engrams* as they are known, stay with us for many years. For instance, even if we have not ridden a bicycle for many years, we are still capable of doing so without falling off. Engrams also set a neuromuscular pattern in our brain, so certain movements become habitual. These habits may not affect us for years. The problems occur when we change a habit and attempt a different movement.

Our pattern of movement, then, becomes our physical "safety zone." Even if we know we move in an ungainly way (usually because it's been pointed out to us, not because we have noticed it ourselves), we feel it is normal.

For example, walking with slight knock-knees is not a grossly distorted movement. It is, however, noticeable to others. To the person walking this way, the movement seems normal, and the gait feels just as fast and fluid in execution as anyone else's, but it is not how 90 percent of the population walks. If the gait is to be corrected, the inherent pattern of movement requires change. Even though the person who has knock-knees may experience no physical discomfort, there may be reasons to change his or her way of walk-

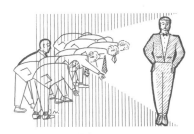

*Figure 2.*
*"Look at the abnormal posture on that guy?"*

## JOHN M.

*John M. could stand normally and outwardly appeared not to have any structural problems. However, he could not touch his toes from a standing position, even after extensive stretching and exercise. He could stretch the hamstrings on his individual legs without problems, as these were quite flexible; it was the lower back that was moderately tight.*

*A decision was made to invert the client, using hanging boots. When relaxed in an inverted position, John M. was found to have a marked rotation of the spine not evident in the normal standing position. After a series of appropriate exercises to counter the imbalance, he was easily able to touch his toes.*

ing, such as to improve speed in a 100-meter race, or to walk as a model down a catwalk.

Similar muscular pulls occur in many of our everyday movements: women who wear high heels walk with a forward tilt, which they correct unconsciously by leaning backward. The result is a forward tilt of the pelvis; the compensation of the backward lean tends to arch and tighten the lower back.

In most cases a realignment of the body's "abnormal" position to one that is normal requires a reeducation of the musculature, assuming there are no structural (skeletal) problems.

From the preceding case study we see that our body will align itself without our knowledge according to its own frame of reference. In this case, the frame of reference is a "squaring" of the torso when standing. Visual images of what is straight and correct alignment are imprinted in our subconscious from what we see around us. We then stand accordingly, even if this is not our "natural" position.

Another example is children who experience growth spurts and outgrow their peers, or girls who develop large breasts at an early age. These young people tend to walk with stooped shoulders to avoid bringing attention to themselves. This action tightens the pectoral group of muscles in the chest, resulting in rounded shoulders or a stooped posture that may be carried into adulthood, even though their peers have caught up in height! As a corrective measure, to avoid future problems in the neck and even the lower back, the muscles in the middle of the back, between the shoulder blades (the rhomboids), would need strengthening and the chest muscles lengthening.

In the example of the woman in high heels, the back muscles are forced to tighten into an arch in order to prevent the body from leaning forward. This can lead to a weakening of the opposing muscles—the abdominals. The weakening of the abdominals and the forward (anterior) tilt of the pelvis lead to tight thighs, or quadriceps (see Figure 3).

The situations I've described are of less concern if they do not cause discomfort. However, many years of repeating the same action can set the muscle into what becomes its normal pattern, and this can eventually lead to more noticeable problems, especially if the person fails to follow a corrective exercise program.

Tightness in one group of muscles invariably indicates a weakness in another, usually opposite, group of muscles. In the high-heel example, the weak area would be the abdominals. However, strengthening the abdominals is not the total solution to the condition. Stretching and lengthening the tight muscles (calves, thighs, psoas) is also of great importance in alleviating the problem. Control of these muscles on a continual basis is important. If the lower back is arched because of weak abdominals, then concentration is required to "pull" the abdominals in, even when standing at a bus stop. Reminding the muscles to do the right thing will eventually lead to a more comfortable,

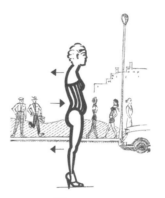

*Figure 3.*
*In those high heels*

correct posture. However, people find it easier to let the body think for itself than to remind it what to do for a few seconds now and then.

Here's a simple activity that can demonstrate how we develop patterns of movement: Fold your arms across your chest, as you would normally do. Next, stretch your hands above your head, then rest them by your side, and now fold your arms the opposite way as quickly as possible. A little confusion occurs here. You may have to focus visually, as well as mentally, on what you are doing. Retraining your thinking to perform the new movement is unusual and requires focus. And tomorrow when you fold your arms, you will automatically revert to the old, set pattern. We do not want to make the extra effort necessary to relearn patterns of movement. Why should we? Everything works well enough, does it not? So leave it alone! As the saying goes, "If it ain't broke don't fix it."

Varying a set pattern, however unnatural the set pattern is, causes confusion both physically and mentally. For a new pattern to become habit takes far longer than we might anticipate. Many people assume that when pain occurs it can be fixed immediately and permanently. In many cases, if the pain is not caused by a sporting injury or an accident, it is the result of an accumulation of incorrect muscle control over a period of time. This gradual buildup of muscle imbalance can later manifest itself in one sudden occurrence: You might be doing something as simple as turning around a little farther than usual in the car seat while driving in reverse, when suddenly your back "gives out." However slight this extra, different movement is, in some cases it is capable of causing extreme pain.

We can see the effects of chronic pain in people all around us. We all know someone who endures pain of some kind, whether it be back pain, neck and shoulder pain, or another type. Pain can be a debilitating "dis-ease" that can lead us to despair of ever finding a "cure."

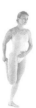

## LOADING THE BODY

Weight training and certain sporting activities, such as tennis and golf, create unbalanced muscle structures purely because of the nature of the action that the muscle is required to undertake. For example, the playing forearm of a world-class squash player would be significantly larger than the nonplaying arm. In our everyday lives, the body is "loaded" by normal gravitational forces and also by unnatural forces such as the lifting of shopping bags or the lifting of weights at the gym. These activities sometimes impose a greater force than the counterforce exerted by the body to sustain a level of equilibrium, resulting in muscle strain and possible injury. For example, lifting or bench-pressing a weight greater than that which the body is capable of sustaining results in an extra strain that leads to torn muscles, because the muscles were commanded to exert a far greater effort than they were capable of adequately supporting.

Our joints endure tremendous forces when we run, climb, jump, bend, twist, arch, push, and pull. Joints affected by these movements include practically every place in the body where a bone comes into contact with another bone. For example, although we commonly think of the joints at the elbow, shoulder, hip, knee, wrist, and ankle as bearing most of the brunt of our activities, even those at the fingers, toes, and spine (the vertebrae) are affected by our patterns of motion.

As I have mentioned, gravity is a major stress on the body. As Isaac Newton said, "To every action, there is an equal and opposite reaction." This is true of every movement we undertake; each of our movements is a counteraction against the gravitational pull of the earth. It is when we make a movement to which the body cannot react comfortably that the weakest joint or muscle may give way, and occasionally even the strongest muscles and joints may overload and strain.

Our skeletal frame is held together by muscles, tendons, and ligaments. We feel overexertion as aching muscles, perhaps after a strenuous aerobics class or a long run. Too much stress or more loading than is comfortable affects not only the muscles but also the tendons and/or ligaments. (Tendons are the connective tissues that attach muscle to bone; ligaments attach bone to bone.) For example, sudden loading and twisting on a skier's knee can tear the cruciate ligaments in the back of the knee, causing him to feel pain in the knee joint.

The direction of the forces that are placed on the joint is also a determining factor in the resultant ache or break of the muscle or bone. In the example of the skier, he could reduce his chances of injury by maintaining flexibility in his hips, knees, and spine. In addition, strength in his thighs, buttocks, and abdominals would give him a greater sense of balance when he's in a forward, bent position. Football players need extra strength to protect their joints because of the extra forces placed on their bodies from all directions. A football player is tackled from the front, back, sides, and other angles, and by different amounts of force, depending on the weight and size and speed of the person performing the tackle.

If a football player were to ski and a skier were to play football, it is clear that further physical conditioning, strengthening, and a change of mental attitude would be required for each to perform the other's sport. Because the muscular and joint stresses of these activities are different, each athlete would ache after an initial training session in the other's sport.

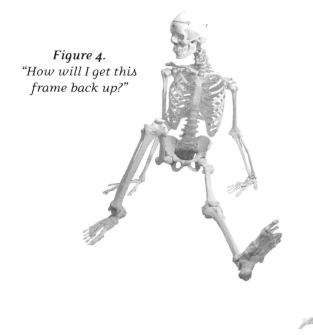

*Figure 4.*
*"How will I get this frame back up?"*

# THE IMPORTANCE OF LEVERS

*"Give me a lever long enough
and I will move the Earth!"*

— ARISTOTLE

In order to understand the concept of stresses or loads on muscle groups, we need to understand the principle of levers and how they relate to the human body. Having this knowledge will help us be aware of how to reduce the strain on certain muscles by physically (and mentally) applying effort from a stronger muscle in order to protect weaker muscles and joints. (Portions of the following discussion of levers and the human body have been adapted from *Fitness Theory and Practice*, 2nd ed. See References.)

Levers are rigid rods that move about a *fulcrum* (also called an *axis* or *pivot point*). Two different types of forces act on the lever: *resistance* (or load) and *effort*. In the human body, the lever is the bone, the fulcrum is the joint, the effort force comes from the muscle, and the resistance force comes from gravity. Resistance may be increased by adding weight or using elastic bands.

There are three basic types of lever systems: first-class, second-class, and third-class (see Figures 5a through 5d). These classes are based on the relative location on the lever of the fulcrum, the effort or applied force, and the resistance force or load. In a *first-class lever system* the fulcrum is located between the applied force and the resistance (for example, a see-saw). Note that in a first-class lever system the effort and the resistance can be equidistant from the fulcrum (Figure 5a), or one can be closer to the fulcrum than the other (Figure 5b). The relative distances from the fulcrum of the effort and the resistance affect the amount of work required to lift the load. In a *second-class lever system* (Figure 5c), the fulcrum is at one end of the lever, the effort is at the opposite end, and the resistance (or load) is in between them. In a *third-class lever system* (Figure 5d), the fulcrum is at one end, the resistance is at the other end, and the applied force is in between them (for example, a human arm bending at the elbow to lift a weight that is held in the hand).

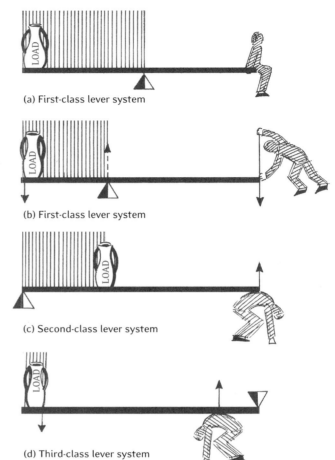

(a) First-class lever system

(b) First-class lever system

(c) Second-class lever system

(d) Third-class lever system

***Figure 5.** The three basic types of lever systems*

Most of the human musculoskeletal system is made up of third-class levers. As noted in the example above, visualize holding a weight in your hand, then bending your elbow to raise the weight (while keeping your upper arm still). The fulcrum or axis is your elbow joint; the applied force is the upward effort of your forearm; and the resistance is the downward force exerted by the weight in your hand. Although more force is required to move an object in a third-class lever system, this system allows for greater speed and range of motion.

The heavier the weight or load (resistance), the more the muscle and surrounding structures are required to work. When the muscle exerts a greater effort than the resistance, the body can

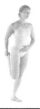

usually lift the weight quite comfortably. As the resistance increases, so, too, does the effort required by the muscle. Although the resistance may not exceed the force exerted by the muscle, the muscle may still strain. Whether and how much it strains depends on the condition of the muscle and the amount of time the external load is applied. The greater the duration, the more likely it is that the muscle will strain.

As the load or resistance applied exceeds the point at which the muscle is able to support the load, the effort exerted by the muscle must be greater than that of the load or the muscle may tear or rupture. This may happen immediately with an extremely heavy load, particularly if the muscle is not warmed up; for example, when a person lifts a very heavy box, the back muscles may become "overloaded" and pull. The same thing may happen if the same weight is constantly applied over a lengthy period of time and the endurance of the muscle is no longer able to contain the stress of the weight; an example of this could be holding a heavy weight at arm's length for a period of time.

We can see how easy it is to strain our bodies by placing forces on them. Our bodies require ongoing conditioning in order to meet the physical demands of everyday living. If we can mentally condition ourselves to perform daily, basic physical-conditioning routines, we will become increasingly mentally capable of enduring the stresses of living. We will have created a beneficial cycle of achievement!

On the other hand, if our bodies are under stress, we tend to feel pain, and this can create a cycle of discomfort. When we feel pain, our body's automatic reaction is to protect the injured area. This manifests itself as a tightening of the muscles around the injury. Thus we restrict the movement of the area for fear of doing more damage. This lack of normal mobility hampers the healing process. When we then attempt a normal movement from that area of the body, without adequate conditioning and rehabilitation, we still feel restricted, with the result being less mobility and even more protection (tightening) of the area.

To overcome this detrimental cycle, it is important for us to understand how our bodies work

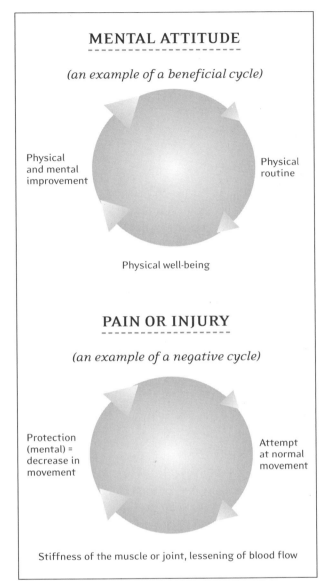

Figure 6. Examples of beneficial and negative cycles

and how they react to various stresses. Properly strengthening and stretching our bodies is a vital part of breaking the cycle. Doing so also assists in the prevention of further injury to the same area and to other parts of the body.

As we become more aware of our body and how it functions, we are more likely to discover hidden quirks and peculiarities. For instance, a client once said that she never realized she had back pain until it went away! We live with many "hidden"

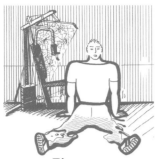

*Figure 7.*
*Lack of exercise =*
*weak muscles*

stresses every day. Our bodies have learned to cope with them. However, our lives would be more fulfilled if we could control many of the subconscious movements we take for granted—either movements that cause twinges (often ignored warnings of things to come) or restrictions that prevent us from doing what we once enjoyed, such as sports, or that simply prevent us from feeling agile and alert as we grow older.

There are no shortcuts to a better body, a new self, or a sense of achieving renewed vigor and vitality at whatever age we choose. We wonder why our bodies "fall apart" as we grow older. If we did not brush our teeth daily, our teeth would eventually decay and fall out. Similarly, if we do not exercise our bodies regularly, using the right techniques, our bodies will also "decay" and "fall apart."

## YOU CAN DO IT!

Imagine an exercise routine that can give you a firmer, flatter stomach, improve your posture, provide you with more energy, may-be make you taller, and even improve your sex life! Imagine an exercise routine that does not involve mindless jumping around to loud, thumping music. Imagine an exercise routine that provides you with the stretching benefits of a yoga class and the strengthening of a gym routine. Imagine an exercise routine that provides you with the control, balance, and strength of a gymnast or a competitive athlete, without a steamy sweat session. Imagine having more stamina at the end of each day.

Now imagine combining all of these benefits into one exercise routine. The Pilates program presented in this book does just that. This is a routine that will change your life and your attitude toward your own body. This is a routine that can give you

increased vitality, make you feel years younger, and improve your posture—all while toning flabby muscles. This is a routine than can eliminate nagging back pain and help you enjoy a better sex life.

The style of Pilates presented in this book is based on the eight extremely sound principles that form the foundation of the original Pilates method. They are presented in Chapter 2. It is important to remember that the original method was devised almost ninety years ago. Some Pilates traditionalists, though brilliant in the application of Joseph Pilates' approach, have been reluctant to vary the original teachings. But today we live a

### FIONA R.

*Fiona R., a middle-aged woman attending a normal gym, approached an instructor and mentioned that she had a "weak back." Without questioning her about the history of her condition, or the amount of exercise or warm-up she'd done prior to her consultation with him, the instructor placed her on a weighted back-extension machine and asked her to complete three sets of ten repetitions, in order to strengthen her back. Before completing her first set, she complained that her lower back now hurt even worse. With the added resistance of the weights on the upper part of the back, the effort required to extend the back became greater than the lower-back muscles could sustain, which resulted in the increased pain. However, if her abdominal muscles had been strong enough to support her lower-back muscles, the effort required by the back muscles would have been lessened.*

*Her case wasn't unusual. In many cases of "weak" lower backs (usually a description of pain in the area), it's really the abdominal muscles that are too weak. In this case, Fiona R. should initially have been referred to a health-care practitioner for evaluation before beginning any loaded back exercises.*

very different lifestyle than we did almost ninety years ago, and we have additional knowledge of human anatomy and the body's ways of moving. This book couples a foundation firmly routed in the Pilates method with the knowledge gained over the last several decades.

Joe Pilates' techniques have evolved, and with that evolution has come a more exact, precise, and athletic approach to the method—the approach described in this book. The original balletic approach to Pilates has held the method in good stead with dancers, ex-dancers, and others influenced by dance. Yet it is important to incorporate our knowledge of the different movements required by a variety of body types. Therefore, we have not used professional models for the poses in this book, but rather ordinary individuals who are Pilates converts.

The exercises described in this book have been refined and enhanced over a period of eighteen years, taking into account the athlete in every person. This does not mean that the program is for

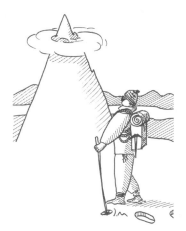

**Figure 8.**
*It may seem daunting now, but not when you look down from the top!*

athletes alone. It has been carefully designed and organized for skill levels ranging from basic to advanced, for those who are injured and those who are supremely fit, for those of any age and any ability. It is for the athlete in all of us.

Pilates is a safe, no-impact exercise routine that stretches and strengthens all the major muscle groups in a logical sequence, without neglecting the smaller, weaker muscles. It can be customized for the individual requirements of any body. In the following pages I have provided the most comprehensive guide to the exercises so that many people may experience the benefits of Pilates. However, the book is no substitute for a qualified, experienced Pilates instructor or a studio registered with the Pilates Institute of Australasia or with an affiliated organization outside of Australia.

As you will discover, the exercises at first are a challenge, both physically and mentally. But if you persist, you will find that you can achieve fantastic results. Persistence is the key.

If you think you can do it, you can!

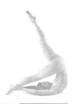

# Mental Control over Physical Movement

The science of
Contrology
disproves that
prevalent and all-
too-trite saying
"you're only as old
as you feel."

— J. Pilates

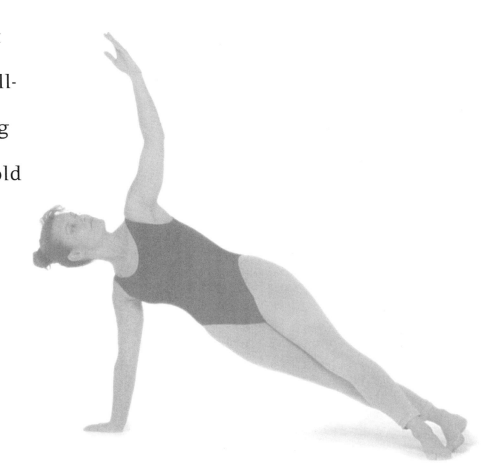

# THE INEVITABLE AGING PROCESS

------------------------------------------

*Life is a challenge!*

— A. Menezes

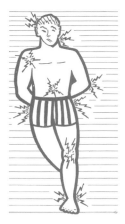

*Figure 9.*
*"Ouch!"*

It has often been stated that if exercise came in a pill, it would be the most prescribed drug in the Western world. The best formula for the reduction and avoidance of muscle pain is not magic, and it doesn't come in a pill, but it is simple: exercise, mobilize, visualize. Keeping the joints supple without putting stress on the musculoskeletal structure is as good, and as simple, a tonic as any. The secret lies not in the achievement of flexibility at any cost but in the physical control and mental understanding of the movement being performed.

Do keep in mind that exercising an injured part of the body or a specific muscle should always be done under the supervision of a qualified exercise-oriented practitioner or qualified Pilates instructor.

Before allowing our bodies to get to the late stage of deterioration depicted in Figure 9, we are sent the occasional warning signals—the odd muscle cramp here, the unusual twinge or minor ache there. We tend to ignore these minor signs, thinking, "Oh! It's nothing. It will take care of itself." If only it would. We assume, even if we have been sitting down all day for years, that if we just do a quick jog around the block (as long as we lack any signs of an impending heart attack), we are as fit as a fiddle and can play a three-hour game of competitive tennis the next day. We consider the jog our self-assessment fitness test—and we passed! We tell ourselves that as long as we don't suffer any serious aftereffects, we must have the athletic capability of a teenager.

With minimal warming up and less-than-adequate stretching, we then push our bodies to their limits. We would be surprised if we didn't ache the following day. "This must be good," we say to ourselves. "I must have worked my muscles really well." And then we remain inactive until the following week—or longer.

The infrequency with which many of us tend to our bodies is scandalous. We often care for our cars better than we care for the far more complex "machines" of our bodies, with so many thousands more delicate parts. Anything more serious than the occasional ache or pain and we shuffle off to the doctor or health practitioner, who prescribes a concoction of tablets whose names we cannot pronounce, or treats the affected area, which has been aching for days, in under an hour. We feel better and assume the problem is fixed for good.

Unfortunately, for most of us this is our body's first warning of the beginning of the decay process. This "decay" does not necessarily take place throughout the entire body at the same time. It could be a knee problem here, a neck strain there.

Why is it that we were once able to get through a high-impact aerobic session with such ease, yet after we go a few years without much strenuous activity, we find that we are suddenly starting to fall apart? The reason is simple. The wear and tear that the body and joints have been subjected to for many years is just beginning to manifest itself. Combine these ingredients with the lack of a safe, regular stretching and conditioning program, and we have a recipe for immobility, discomfort, and, altogether, pain.

In years gone by, we were capable of pushing our bodies without too much warming up. And our bodies were able to withstand that pressure. Young muscles can easily cope with spontaneous strenuous activity. Unfortunately, we believe we have an endless source of

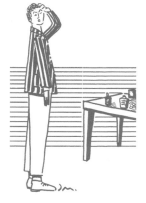

*Figure 10.*
*Jim the Junkie—*
*deciding which*
*tablet will keep*
*him the fittest!*

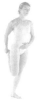

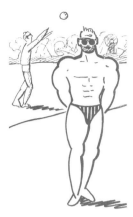

*Figure 11.*
*This body is*
*as young as ever.*

youthful vigor without having to work to maintain it or to "keep those batteries charged." On a pleasant, sunny afternoon when we're hanging out with friends we still feel capable of over-reaching for that elusive return of the soccer ball, tennis ball, or volleyball. Ouch! Too late. The damage is done. We feel a sharp pain in the back, hamstring, or shoulder, yet we continue to play, because we feel we are fit (or we wish to appear so to those around us). The pain is bearable. We retire to bed and trust that a good night's rest will see us well in the morning. Morning arrives—and we cannot move!

Such signs of aging do not affect only us mere mortals. We see them in professional athletes, too. Even ballet dancers, who seem the epitome of flexibility and fitness to most of us, acquire creaky hip, knee, and ankle joints. No one escapes the onset of old age. However, there are solutions for coping with the onset of physical senility so that we can enjoy a more pain-free and fulfilling life.

## FIND YOUR FOCUS

*By reawakening thousands and*
*thousands of otherwise ordinary*
*dormant muscle cells, Contrology*
*correspondingly reawakens thousands*
*and thousands of dormant brain cells,*
*thus activating new areas and stimulating*
*further the functioning of the mind.*

— J. PILATES

When our bodies fail us, we are somewhat surprised. An injury that lays us low, especially if it hospitalizes us, can be emotionally devastating. The grief process we go through after being immobilized by an injury can parallel that of losing a loved one.

During our physical rehabilitation, many of us pay considerable attention to the precise details of what is required to get us back on track, sometimes to the point of obsession. We become knowledgeable about muscles, injury, and the curing of our particular complaint. Most of us are capable of achieving positive results after injury because we are determined to overcome our affliction. We become mentally focused on our goal. But this focus can be used to prevent injuries from happening in the first place. It can be used to gain greater control over weak muscle groups. It can be used to improve our performance in whatever sport or movement we desire.

## DEVELOPING A "THINKING BODY"

*Contrology begins with*
*mind control over muscles.*

— J. PILATES

Concentrating on the precision of our physical movements makes us mentally alert. This takes practice and repetition. We need to develop a "thinking body," one that is eventually able to control movements, however demanding, with precision, control, and fluidity, without our having to think consciously about the demands of the movement.

To develop a thinking body, we need to understand the body itself: the major muscle groups and their functions, and how they affect physical outcomes. To that end, I have provided the following list of terms. My purpose is to give you a broad understanding of these concepts without being too clinical. Many of you who have suffered injuries or who otherwise have a working knowledge of physiology and movement will already be familiar with these terms.

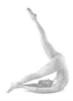

# MOVEMENT TERMS

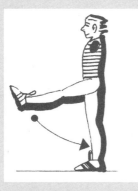

**EXTENSION**
means lengthening out
or straightening.

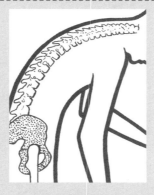

**FLEXION**
means folding or
bending. Flexors of the
toes curl the toes.

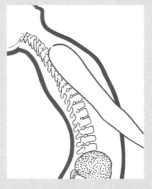

**HYPEREXTENSION**
means extending more
than 180 degrees.

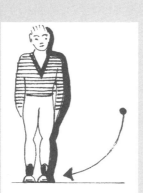

**ADDUCTION**
means movement that
draws inward (toward the
midline of the body).

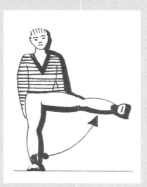

**ABDUCTION**
means movement that
draws away (from the
midline of the body).
Adductors and abductors
oppose one another.

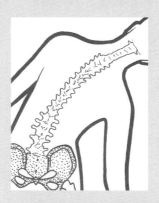

**LATERAL FLEXION**
is a side bend of
the body.

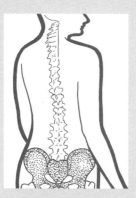

**ROTATION**
means movement
around the central axis
of a lever.

# ANATOMICAL TERMS

**TENDON:** elastic connective tissue
that connects muscle to bone.

**LIGAMENT:** nonelastic connective
tissue that connects bone to bone.

**LORDOSIS:** the hyperextension of
the normal curve in the lumbar or
cervical spine.

**KYPHOSIS:** the forward flexion of
the normal thoracic curve of the spine.

**SCOLIOSIS:** lateral curvature of
the spine.

**SUPINE:** on the back.

**PRONE:** on the stomach.

**RANGE OF MOTION/MOVEMENT
(ROM):** the degree to which a limb
may comfortably move around a joint
without affecting other parts of
the body.

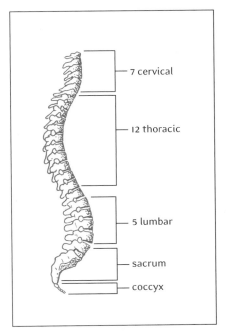

*Figure 12. The vertebral column*

The skeletal system is comprised of 226 bones. The important areas of mobilization, in combination with the muscles, include all the major joints. These joints are separated into two major categories:

1. Hinge joints: for example, ankle, knee, and elbow.

2. Rotational joints (ball and socket): hip, shoulder, wrist.

The entire skeleton is held together by muscles, tendons, ligaments, and connective tissue. Without the skeleton and these other tissues, we would simply fall to the floor because of gravity. The skeleton has several important functions:

1. It acts as a framework to support the softer parts of the body.

2. It protects the more delicate areas of the body, such as the brain, heart, lungs, and spinal cord.

3. It helps to produce blood cells in the bones, which contain marrow.

4. Together with the contraction of the muscles, it allows us to move.

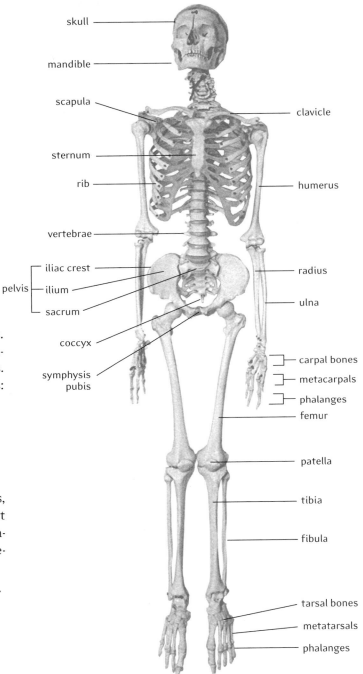

*Figure 13. The skeleton*

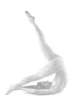

*Figure 14. The major muscles—front and back*

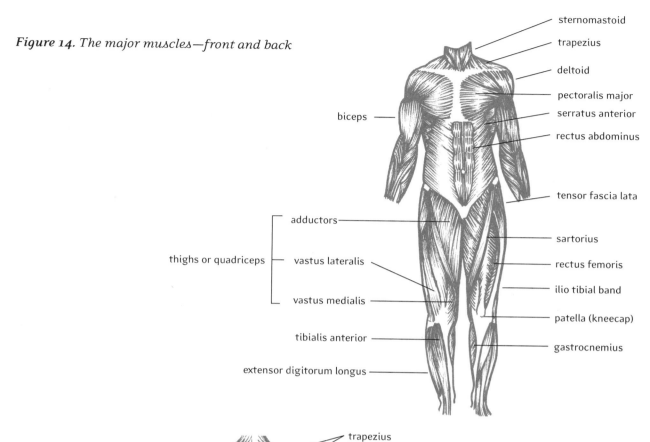

sternomastoid
trapezius
deltoid
pectoralis major
biceps
serratus anterior
rectus abdominus
tensor fascia lata
adductors
sartorius
thighs or quadriceps
vastus lateralis
rectus femoris
ilio tibial band
vastus medialis
patella (kneecap)
tibialis anterior
gastrocnemius
extensor digitorum longus

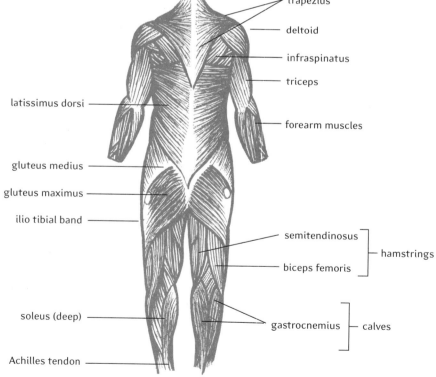

trapezius
deltoid
infraspinatus
triceps
latissimus dorsi
forearm muscles
gluteus medius
gluteus maximus
ilio tibial band
semitendinosus
hamstrings
biceps femoris
soleus (deep)
gastrocnemius
calves
Achilles tendon

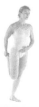

## THE EIGHT PRINCIPLES OF THE PILATES METHOD

To understand Joseph Pilates' method, we first need to learn the principles behind the technique. Being ignorant of the essentials is akin to attempting to drive a car without the engine: You may cruise down the hills, but driving becomes extremely hard work when you reach the uphills!

In Pilates, the manner in which the exercises are performed is of far greater importance than the number of repetitions or the amount of exertion applied to the movements. *Quality is superior to quantity.* In fact, to master a simple movement is sometimes more difficult than to force the body to perform strenuous tasks. By combining application and dedication to the basic principles, you can more easily achieve your desired results. It is the mind's subconscious control over habitual movements that needs to be altered in order for us to progress above and beyond our standard capabilities.

The eight principles are:

1. Concentration
2. Centering
3. Breathing
4. Control
5. Precision
6. Flowing Movement
7. Isolation
8. Routine

(Joseph Pilates created the first six principles. We have added the last two as they increase the challenge for the participant.)

These principles may at first appear simple and logical in their individual parts. But it can be challenging to remember all of them at the same time when performing even a basic exercise. When you first begin the program, focusing on even two of the principles may require some effort. Slowly, as you are able to master one principle at a time with some of the simpler exercises, you will discover the enormous effect that even a slight variation in the movement can have.

As we begin to master the exercises, we become capable of achieving more. This may take some time. We continue to perform the exercises that we find relatively easy, with the goal of incorporating more challenging variations of the same exercises. As we progress we discover at the end of a session that our energy levels have increased. The days do not seem as long, and we look forward to physical and mental challenges without regarding them as insurmountable problems. We sleep better, we awake more refreshed, and our physical and mental reflexes are more highly tuned.

As mentioned earlier, Frederich von Schiller, an eighteenth-century German philosopher, once said, "It is the mind itself which builds the body." With Joseph Pilates' techniques, we are not only exercising our body but also simultaneously exercising our mind.

Let's look at each of the eight principles more closely.

## 1. CONCENTRATION

*Concentrate on the correct movements each time you exercise, lest you do them improperly and thus lose all the vital benefits of their value.*

— J. Pilates

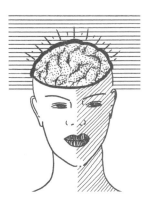

*Figure 15. Concentration makes life easier.*

To focus on muscles as they move is a challenging task to master. The body resists following what the mind wants it to do. Our initial movements may be awkward and jerky. Once we achieve continual mental focus, we realize that simple movements are actually quite complex.

The first step in learning to concentrate is realizing that the position of every part of the body is of great importance, and that all of our movements and positions are interconnected. When we walk or run, or when we reach for a cup of coffee, the positioning of the foot or arm is both influenced and affected by the correct alignment of the body. For that reason, concentration is required when following each of the other seven principles. You will discover that in order to accomplish even the simplest exercises your mind needs to focus on small movements.

Achieving this level of concentration offers benefits in all realms of life: clarity of thought; better mental focus leading to increased mental energy; increased ability to handle difficult situations more calmly and positively; fresh approaches to new and unusual conditions; etc.... Over time, like the benefits of the exercises themselves, the meditative effect of continual concentration seeps into the subconscious, and the entire body and mind are more energized after the exercise routine. As we correctly perform the movements, we find that we are unable to think of other things that have happened during the day.

## THE IMPORTANCE OF POSITION

*Tennis players do most of their abdominal strength work by performing crunches with the knees bent. When they stand up, their abdominal muscles are more lengthened and have less strength than they did in the position in which they were worked. As a result, when they serve, and their abdominal muscles are at a full stretch, there is no strength from their center to perform the movement efficiently and effectively. That means the majority of the force for the serve comes from the shoulder and arm. If the abdominals were developed so that they remained strengthened when at a full stretch, the body's center could be brought into play and the serve would be more effective. The same principle applies to most sports and other activities.*

Again, to concentrate on the entire body at the same time as it performs complex movements is a formidable challenge and takes time, so don't be discouraged if your initial efforts seem fruitless. Concentration is a skill you will acquire as the method becomes more familiar. As your movements begin to achieve a level of precision, the results become noticeable.

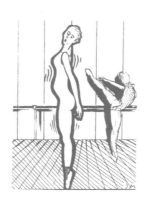

*Figure 16. Dancer with potbelly*

## 2. CENTERING

The abdominal area is often described as the second spine. It is the powerhouse of the anatomy. Pilates defined the body's center as the area between the ribs and the hips at both the front and the back of the torso. In this book we define the body's center as also including the sides of the torso. A strong center is important to maintaining good control and balance in the body as a whole. It provides assistance for movements both slow and fast, such as balancing on a beach ball or sprinting one hundred meters.

Imagine a ballet dancer standing on one leg *en pointe* (on the toes), with the other leg pointed to the ceiling and her arms above her head. Now imagine if she had loose abdominals (or, worse, a potbelly)! She would fall over instantly.

The center is the pivotal point of the body. All strength movements emanate from this area. In karate, the *ki* (meaning life force or energy) comes from the solar plexus. The efforts of movement, force, balance, and strength come from the center.

Note that abdominal control is different from abdominal strength. (However, the former does rely on the latter.) It is preferable to have control. In many workout routines, most of the abdominal strength is achieved by performing crunches, situps, or some other manner of forward contraction or flexion of the body. This limits the control of the

*Figure 17.* How to find your B-Line

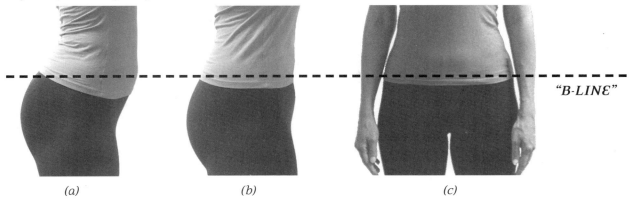

*(a)*             *(b)*             *(c)*             "B-LINE"

abdominal muscles and most of their strength to that position where the abdominal contraction takes place: a forward curved position of the torso. Abdominal strength provides support, while abdominal control provides fluidity of movement from the center.

### The B-Line

The concept of the B-Line is a new approach to abdominal control. The emphasis of the B-Line is on the exactness of the movement and how best to engage the lower abdominals. The B-Line, together with correct foot placement, is the foundation of good posture. (See "The Tripod Position," in Chapter 3.)

To find your B-Line, do the following:

- Stand upright, with your feet hip distance apart.

- Draw the abdominals as close to the spine as possible and breathe normally.

What do you feel? You may notice several things:

1. The area drawing to the spine is generally the navel, or the middle and upper abdominals, with some engagement (connection) of the lower abdominals.

2. The pelvis may be tucked to provide a feeling of flattening the back (this especially happens when lying on the floor or standing against a wall).

3. The knees may bend slightly or the shoulders round. The ribs may drop slightly to the hips.

4. The buttocks may be clenched.

5. Breathing may be somewhat restricted, with a feeling of forcing the breath into the lungs.

6. There is generally little or no feeling of abdominal contraction in the area below the navel.

Now, abolish all thoughts of drawing the navel to the spine!

Stand as before and relax. Now, do the following, without clenching the buttocks, tucking the pelvis, or dropping the shoulders:

1. With your finger, trace a straight line from the top of one hipbone (anterior superior iliac spine) to the other. You may notice that the line is in front of the hipbones (Figure 17a).

2. Go to the center of this line (two to three inches below the belly button) and press with your fingers. Now draw the stomach away from the fingers. Press further and draw in again. (The term *B-Line* comes from visualizing that the line lies *behind* the line of the hipbones.)

When was the last time you felt these lower-abdominal muscles working?

This is the B-Line. *Maintain it for the rest of your life!* (We will use the term *B-Line* throughout the book, but women can think of this as the "Bikini line" and men can think of this as the "Belt line.") Initially, you may feel some mild discomfort in the lower back. This will diminish as your body becomes used to its new position. You may notice that you are standing a little more upright. Your breathing may still feel restricted. Be sure to breathe as described in the section below on breathing.

### The B-Line in Action

Stand up out of your chair. You may notice that your upper body first leaned forward over your knees, before you came to the standing position. Take a seat again, and now engage your B-Line before you rise up out of the chair. You may have noticed that you stood up without leaning forward so far, and your back may have felt more supported.

### The B-Line Core and Pelvic Floor

The B-Line Core is a new concept in Pilates and also in physical therapy and other forms of movement. The idea behind the B-Line Core is to provide even more support for the core abdominal muscles, especially when the body is moving outside of the range of linear movements. Engaging the B-Line Core strengthens the abdominals from the back and sides. Up until now all abdominal work has been described as working from the front to the back.

### How to Find Your B-Line Core and Pelvic Floor

#### THE B-LINE CORE

Standing upright, imagine replacing the area between your ribs and hips with a very large apple. Remove the core from the apple and throw it away. You are now left with a hollow cylinder in the middle of the apple (which is roughly in front of your spine). Now, starting from the muscles in the back, squeeze the hollow cylinder from all sides until it disappears. You should feel the lower-back muscles (lumbar multifidis) and the side muscles (obliques) drawing in tightly, and then the front abdominal

section—this is the B-Line Core. Now engage the B-Line (lower abs) strongly and you will feel the pelvic floor start to engage. The pelvic floor is the bottom of this hollow cylinder and the diaphragm is the top.

#### THE PELVIC FLOOR

Once you have engaged your B-Line Core, imagine placing the apple in an elevator and closing the doors. Now take the elevator to the second floor and hold it there for ten seconds. Then take it to the third floor and hold it there for another ten seconds. Next take it to the fourth floor and hold it there for twenty seconds. You will notice that you are, in effect, "lifting" the muscles of the pelvic floor. Practice doing this daily to keep the pelvic floor muscles working. Always make sure to squeeze the Core before the B-Line.

Another way to engage the B-Line Core is by placing the fingers on the sides of the body just above the hip bones (not touching them) with the thumbs placed on the back muscles. Now draw in away from your thumbs first and then in from the fingers on your sides. Now squeeze the bottom of the Core up to your rib cage. Doing so should strongly engage the pelvic floor while also supporting the Core stabilization muscles.

Men should understand that they, too, have a pelvic floor. By engaging these muscles on a regular basis, both men and women can minimize problems such as incontinence. Doing so will also tremendously help women to reengage these important muscles after childbirth, in order to help prevent a prolapse of the uterus.

## 3. BREATHING

*To breathe correctly you must completely exhale and inhale, always trying very hard to "squeeze" every atom of impure air from your lungs in much the same manner that you would wring every drop of water from a wet cloth.*

— J. Pilates

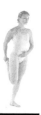

Breathing is the most important physical principle to refine before attempting an exercise or movement. Breathing has three major functions:

1. To carry nutrients to all parts of the body, thereby charging the whole body with more energy.

2. To carry away wastes for elimination from the body.

3. To increase stamina.

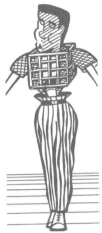

*Figure 18. Restricted breathing*

Wastes can produce restrictions within the body's system. These can be various, such as tightness and restricted movement in joints, tiredness, headaches, and pain. This is not to say that breathing on its own can cure these conditions—it cannot. But, combined with the other principles, it can certainly lead to greater well-being. Drinking the required quantity of water (eight glasses per day) to assist in waste elimination also helps greatly in achieving this goal. It has also been suggested that adequate water consumption can improve flexibility of the muscles.

As we have all seen at the gym, people often hold their breath at the most crucial part of an exercise, when releasing it could be most beneficial. You have probably been guilty of this yourself without realizing it. When we do this, we put our bodies under an enormous amount of physical tension, especially in the upper thoracic and cervical areas (neck and shoulders).

When we hold the breath while exercising, we create a situation similar to that of pressure building inside a pressure cooker. As a result, we waste energy and exert unnecessary effort. The outcome is a less-than-efficient use of the working muscles.

Try this simple exercise. Breathe in to raise your arms above your head. Hold your breath as you lower your arms back down to your sides and simultaneously imagine squeezing oranges in your armpits. Can you feel the tension in your neck and shoulders? Now repeat the same exercise, but as you lower your arms gradually release the breath in a long sigh. Can you feel how much more relaxing this is?

You will notice that throughout the text I have used the phrase "breathe in *to* raise your arms" (or raise your leg, or make any other movement), rather than "breathe in *as you* raise your arms" (or make whatever movement). This seemingly small modification has a significant effect on core (abdominal) control and its engagement in preparation for the exercise. As a simple exercise to follow the one above, imagine you have a weight in your hand, and breathe in *as you* raise your arm. Now repeat the movement, but breathe in *to* raise your arm. Can you feel the difference in establishing core muscle connection? When you breathe in *to* raise your arms, you experience almost a bracing feeling during the movement.

Breathing properly offers other benefits as well. Consider the fact that there are two ways to improve your stamina:

- Cardiovascular workouts (such as running or bike riding).

- Changing your breathing technique.

Correct breathing for the style of Pilates described in this book, Aussie Pilates, should be performed with the following in mind:

1. Keep the neck and shoulders relaxed; hunching causes neck tension.

2. Allow the breath to flow: don't hold your breath at any point.

3. Breathe in through the nose (into the chest) for a slow count of five, without allowing the shoulders to lift. (Try this in front of a mirror, keeping an eye on your shoulders.)

4. Without stopping, breathe out of the mouth with a loud sigh for a slow count of five. Drop the jaw wide and do not purse the lips into any shape. (Breathing out through the teeth or through a tight jaw increases the tension in the neck, jaw, and face.) We call this the "ocean breath out." It sounds like an ocean wave hitting the beach, loud at first and then slowly tapering off at the end. This sound tells you (and the instructor, if applicable) that you are breathing correctly. Once you have gotten used to this kind of breathing, you are able to focus on the important elements of the exercises you're doing.

5. If you find it difficult to breathe while holding in your B-Line Core, breathe into your upper back (shoulder blades) and armpits. Imagine inflating balloons in these areas (see Figure 19). In the exercise descriptions we will mention breathing into the armpits; remember that this also implies breathing into the upper back.

After some practice you may find that your breathing capacity has increased by 20 percent or more, simply by changing your breathing technique and without having to run around the block several times! Try this method of breathing, along with engaging the B-Line Core, in the following exercise.

### Breathing Exercises

Sit down on the floor with your legs comfortably crossed in front of you. Sit as upright as possible, as if your lower back were being supported by a wall, with no gaps between your tailbone and the wall. Do not lean into the wall. Place your hands snugly just below your navel. Without hunching the shoulders, take a five-count breath in through the nose, and then ocean breathe out of the mouth. You may notice that on the breath in you felt the stomach move outward, and on the breath out it went down.

Now repeat the same exercise, except before you breathe in, press your hands very firmly on the B-Line below the navel, pressing against your lower abdominals and toward your spine, and keep them there. Now breathe into your chest. You will find that this is quite difficult to achieve without the hands moving at all. You may also find that the breath into the chest is quite restricted and that there is a slight sensation of "choking" the breath into your chest.

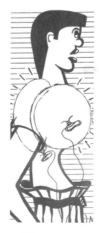

*Figure 19. Breathing "into the back"*

This happens when we become less active because our breathing capacity reduces as the muscles between our ribs, the intercostals, tighten. If we return to our usual level of exercise after a long break, we find that before long we are gasping for breath. As we do less abdominal work, we tend to breathe more into the stomach and thus loosen the abdominal muscles. This is why we feel a choking, restricted sensation when breathing in while holding our abdominals tight.

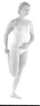

Endurance, or stamina, is the body's ability to perform better over a greater length of time with less stress and fatigue. By controlling your breathing and expanding your lung capacity, you can achieve greater stamina. Many people think that only aerobic activity can increase stamina. However, deeper, controlled breathing, combined with even "low-grade," or nonaerobic, physical activity, is also capable of increasing stamina. As you achieve a certain level of fitness, increase the repetitions without resting. Over a period of time, performing more repetitions, even with ease, will increase muscle endurance and tone. After several weeks of following the principles of breathing and abdominal control outlined here, people have reported increased stamina when doing what was once a strenuous half-hour walk.

If you practice controlled, slow, deep breathing while exercising, you will become accustomed to breathing in this way, so that it will become the norm even when you are at rest. This is less stressful on the body as a whole and can also lower your resting heart rate, which can be a determining factor in your longevity.

Here is a simple technique for overcoming the previously mentioned tightness in the chest. Kneel on the floor with your bottom on your heels. Now lower your chest to your thighs and rest your forehead on the floor (or on cushions if that is more comfortable). Wrap your arms around your torso, placing your hands as high up on your back, on the ribs, as you can without creating any tension in the neck or shoulder area. In this position it would be fairly difficult to take a deep breath into the chest or abdominals, as they are pressed against your thighs. Now breathe into your hands. This has the same effect as breathing into the upper back. Avoid breathing into the chest or abdominals. Practice breathing this way for ten breaths in and out.

### General Breathing Rules

I have created several breathing rules to follow when performing any exercise, whether Pilates or otherwise. (Some exceptions exist to the rules, which I will point out as they occur.) The purposes of the rules are:

- To protect the back;
- To increase stamina;
- To reduce the strain from overexertion.

Here are the rules:

1. When lying on the back (supine), with the arms or the legs moving from a vertical position *away from* the center of the body, ocean breathe out. When the arms or the legs move vertically *toward* the center, breathe in. At all times, maintain the B-Line Core. (When the arms move overhead, also "flatten" the rib cage to support the thoracic [middle] spine; this will reduce any overlifting of the lower back.)

2. When the arms or legs move laterally (out to the sides) away from the median (the midline of the body), breathe in. For example, when performing "flies" (lying on the back with the arms to the ceiling and opening the arms outward), breathe in. Ocean breathe out as they come back to the center.

3. When lying in the side position or on the stomach (prone), if any part of the body is lifted against gravity, squeeze the B-Line Core, and ocean breathe out. Breathe in when lowering to the floor. (However, see the "important exception," below.)

   *Important exception:* When lying prone and lifting the torso, breathe in! This greatly reduces the stress and pressure on the lower back.

4. When on all fours (hands and feet/knees), when drawing the limbs away the center or median, breat in. closing toward the center, keep the navel rmly to the spine and ocean breathe out. Fo xample, see Leg Pull Prone (Exercise 54

5. When contracting (curling forward) or rotating the torso, ocean breathe ou .

### Exercise

Lie on your back on the floor with your knees bent and feet flat on the floor, and your hands placed by your sides, palms upward. Extend one leg into the air, and slowly lower this leg away from you, breathing out. (For those with stronger abdominals, try this exercise with both legs in the air.) If you attempt to breathe in while performing this movement you will feel the back arching.

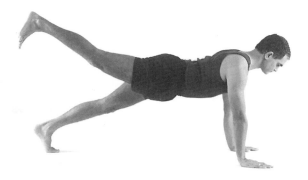

*Figure 20. Breathe in on the leg lift.*

The same can be done with the arms in the air, stretching them toward the floor above the head. As you lower the arms away from your center, you may notice one of two things. You actually want to breathe in, but doing so will cause the upper back to arch as the ribs lift to the ceiling. Now ocean breathe out to repeat the same movement, making sure to maintain the B-Line Core and flattening the rib cage to the floor. You will feel greater core control and better stability in the upper back.

## 4. CONTROL

*Ideally, our muscles should obey our will. Reasonably, our will should not be dominated by the reflex actions of our muscles.*

— J. Pilates

Once the first three principles have been practiced and mastered as well as possible, the next principle, control, can be more easily applied. Control is essential in preventing injuries. Maintaining control of every movement takes concentration, effort, and awareness of what the rest of the body is doing at the same time. Control also involves integrating the previous three principles.

Whether the movements involve simply lengthening the neck and maintaining that position in order to reduce cervical lordosis (an arch in the neck), or whether it is a larger movement, such as a *grande ronde de jambe* in classical dance, the degree of control required may be the same. When someone initially practices these movements, it takes effort and concentration to perfect them to the best of the person's ability. Repetition, dedication, and application improve the degree of control and the perfection of the movement.

Uncontrolled, "automatic" movements, such as performing rapid lat pull-downs (pulling a weight downward and behind the head, with arms out to the sides, to work the latissimus dorsi muscles) can lead to injury if incorrect muscles are used and incorrect posture is enforced. The action becomes mindless. Without concentration and control, the body's stronger muscles will tend to do all the work (and stay stronger), and the weaker, usually flabby muscles will tend to remain relatively unused and therefore weak.

It is gaining control over weaker parts of the body that improves their strength and performance.

---

### SUE P.

*Sue P., a sprinter who attended our Body Control Pilates studios, used to come out of the starting blocks with a "stammering" start—very small steps—until she got into her proper stride. She felt she was losing a fraction of a second as a result, and therefore winning fewer races. When she did the initial work to correct an imbalance in the pelvic area, her times improved. With more specific pelvic-stabilization work, she gained better control and strength in the pelvic area and no longer stammered out of the blocks.*

Control does not necessarily mean a reduction in performance. Initially, as you learn to gain control while doing a certain movement, some performance may be compromised. But when you have perfected the movement, the greater control will allow you to do it more quickly and to exceed your previous levels of performance.

## 5. PRECISION

*Correctly executed and mastered to the point of subconscious reaction, these exercises will reflect grace and balance in your routine activities.*

— J. PILATES

Precision, or exactness, of movement leads to more graceful movements. We see this with classical ballet dancers, who are required to fine-tune their bodies in order to achieve exactness in a simple or complex series of jumps, *ports de bras,* or *pliés,* as well as in gymnasts, who require perfect balance and control when performing on the balance beam or parallel bars. When all these movements are performed in a group, as in synchronized swimming, we can see the beauty, grace, style, and apparent effortlessness that result from precise actions.

Precision requires focus (back to that essential principle of concentration) and mental feedback (visualizing and understanding what the perfect movement is). Our bodies require this feedback to let us know that we are achieving results. It is usually very difficult to obtain this feedback when working weaker muscle groups, because the stronger ones tend to take on most of the workload.

Precision requires controlled action, without which the movement becomes sloppy and aesthetically unappealing. The space within which you move and perform various physical activities also determines, and is determined by, precision.

Precision of movement not only requires correct placement of the body before commencing an exercise or movement, but also regulating the speed with which the movement is performed in relation to other parts of the body. For example, if an exercise requires the movement of your arm above the head as you ocean breathe out, the movement should be synchronized so that the last part of the exhalation coincides with the reach of the arm above the head. If more breath is expelled at the beginning of the movement, so that you are holding your breath for the last 20 percent of the arm's travel, precision of movement may not be achieved. The exercise then becomes stressful rather than flowing and coordinated.

## 6. FLOWING MOVEMENT

*Contrology is designed to give you suppleness, natural grace, and skill that will be unmistakably reflected in [all you do].*

— J. PILATES

When muscles are in continual (flowing) motion, they are being toned. When there is no control (no toning "connection" or "engagement"), they are being underutilized. In broad terms, if you are not toning a muscle, you are "flabbing" it.

Fluidity of movement while exercising leads to fluidity of movement when not exercising. Conscious muscular control through all ranges of movement (ROMs) will help eliminate stiff, jerky movements. It is in the extreme ranges of movement that less control is likely to occur, as muscles tend to be weaker in elongated positions. As a result, there is less flowing movement.

For example, when you extend a leg or an arm to kick or punch, the fast movement at the extremity (end of range) can produce a "snapping" effect in the knee or elbow joint. Continuous repetitions of this action can result in pain in the joint. The snapping of the joint is also an indication that the muscles are in less control than you might think.

This sharp movement can and should be eliminated to reduce any long-term wearing effect on the joint. If it is caused by hyperextension of the joint, then extension should be done only to the point where the joint is "unlocked" (not noticeably bent). To a person with hyperextension, the joint would feel quite bent. However, from a normal visual perspective, the limbs would appear straight.

Stiff movements also occur in muscles that are too tight. We often see this with bodybuilders who lift extremely heavy weights. They walk with short, restricted movements. Their biceps muscles are so tight that their arms are continuously bent, giving the appearance of a gorilla's arm posture. Fluid movement may initially require a shortening of overextended muscles (the triceps) and a lengthening of the tight ones (the biceps).

Make your movements continuous, rather than stopping for even a fraction of a second. Continue the movements as if ten repetitions were one, rather than one repetition repeated ten times.

## 7. ISOLATION

*Each muscle may cooperatively and loyally aid in the uniform development of all our muscles.*

— J. PILATES

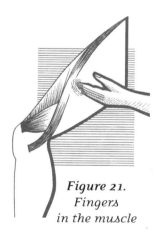

*Figure 21. Fingers in the muscle*

Once you have gained control of a weaker muscle group, you can isolate the muscle more effectively. This allows for greater precision of movement. Isolating a muscle means that you are specifically targeting the muscle you're supposed to be working.

If you have difficulty mentally "feeling" the weak muscles that you're targeting in any given exercise, then follow this suggestion. Press your fingers into the weak/soft/flabby muscle to create a mental connection. For example, when performing Single Leg Circles 1 (Exercise 22), press your fingers into the inner thigh (close to the groin), as shown in Figure 21. Press the fingers against the muscle when taking the leg out to the side, and press the muscle against the fingers when drawing the leg to the center. This will give your mind a better connection to the muscle you want to work, the adductors, as opposed to the quadriceps (thigh) muscle, which you might otherwise tend to overwork. As you press your fingers into the muscle, increasing the pressure usually results in a better response.

If you are unable to obtain the connection, do not despair. It may take several, or even many, attempts for the muscle to respond. Generally, the stronger muscle groups will do the majority of the work in any movement. Concentration alone may not be enough to fire the receptors necessary to engage the weaker muscles that require toning or strength. A muscle does not need to hurt or be sore the next day for you to know that it is working. If the muscle fells firm to the touch when you are doing the exercise, that is a good indication that it is working well.

Once you have gained better control over the weaker muscle, the physical contact of your fingers is no longer required for you to "feel" the muscle working. Successfully isolating the working muscle leads to greater flexibility in the limb, lever, or joint. If you can isolate a part of the body and allow it to move independently of other parts, you are in a better position to introduce more flexibility to that area (assuming you have only muscular, and not structural or bony, restrictions).

## 8. ROUTINE

*Patience and persistence are vital qualities in the ultimate successful accomplishment of any worthwhile endeavor.*

— J. PILATES

Establishing a regular exercise routine, whether it is daily or three times a week, can undoubtedly lead to greater results. Many people ask, "How long will it take me to get fit?" Or, "How often should I exercise?" The answer is relative to the person asking the question. Would you like to become as fit as your next-door neighbor, who may

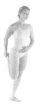

not consider himself fit at all? Or do you go by some other standard?

An established Pilates routine will improve mental and physical conditioning in all individuals. The more you do, the better the result. Your sense of well-being will be vastly improved, and you will see the world through different eyes.

A simple analogy would be playing the piano. Even the world's maestros started from scratch. Their perseverance, dedication, energy, and regular practice made them what they became. The same applies to all activities. One practice session a week will achieve far less than two, three, or four a week.

The workout, including stretches, should take about sixty minutes. At first, working out twice per week is a good effort. Three workouts per week is excellent. Experiencing gradual improvement as you master the exercises will build your confidence in what you are able to achieve physically. You may begin to notice that you're developing a leaner, better defined, and more muscularly balanced physique. I often tell clients to think of this not as exercise (especially when I see them making the all too common mistake of puffing up their cheeks and blowing their breath out through pursed lips during exercise) but simply as movement. Movement that is fluid and unforced, but precise and controlled. I want them to think of these exercises as though they're as natural as a walk in the park, rather than thinking of them as a high-exertion speed walk. Don't be surprised if you fail to see many results for up four weeks. As mentioned earlier, the method works from the inside out. To engage muscles that you never knew even existed takes time. On the other hand, you may be surprised at how soon the results appear; some people see results in as few as five sessions!

When performing the exercises, imagine that they are everyday movements rather than enforced exercises. Imagine walking upstairs and feeling your hamstrings firmly engaging. Imagine picking up a baby or other load and feeling your abdominal muscles supporting your back, or even lifting an object from an awkward position and feeling in total control of all the muscles in your body—all without having to think about these connections happening!

This is what Pilates is about: improved quality of movement that can lead to an improved quality of life. Your life is in your hands. Grasp it with enthusiasm and change the way you think, feel, and react to everything around you.

*Notes*

..................................................

..................................................

..................................................

..................................................

..................................................

..................................................

..................................................

..................................................

..................................................

..................................................

..................................................

..................................................

# 3

# The Importance of Posture

Contrology

develops the

body uniformly,

corrects wrong

postures, restores

physical vitality,

invigorates the

mind, and elevates

the spirit.

— J. Pilates

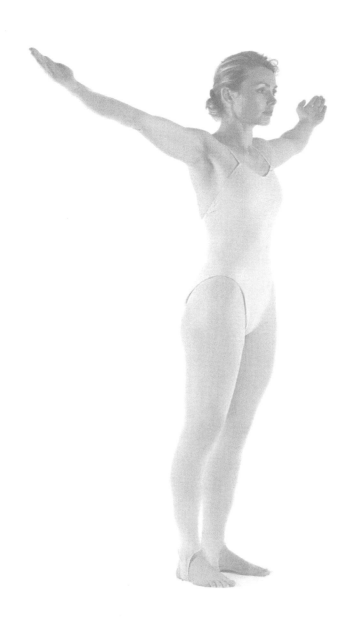

## BODY TYPES

According to the Sheldon classification, there are three basic human body types:

1. *Endomorph:* larger than average, with soft, large abdomen and high shoulders.

2. *Ectomorph:* thin muscles and small bones, with drooped shoulders.

3. *Mesomorph:* large thorax, slender waist, thick abdominal muscles.

The average person lies between the ectomorph and the mesomorph.

## FACTORS INFLUENCING POSTURE

A person with any of the body types can have good or bad posture. Adult posture tends to be dependent on the following:

- Inherited conditions: genetic makeup determines an individual's height, type of bone structure, and so on.

- Habit: from occupational or repetitive movements, muscle function becomes restrictive, altering postural alignment.

- Disease: whether the disease is muscular or structural (as in bone deformity), disease certainly alters one's stance, imposing limitations on one's normal activity.

- Trauma: such as a car accident or breaking a leg.

I have already discussed the effects of gravity on the muscles. They are constantly being pulled downward. Our bodies are required to counter these forces with healthy, strong muscle structures in order to maintain good posture and ward off the effects of strain and injury.

## WHAT IS CORRECT POSTURE?

In order to discuss postural deviation, we need to understand what is meant by normal posture. Imagine a plumb line that goes through your body when you are standing upright:

1. From the side (lateral) view, the plumb line should pass from the top of your skull through the center of your whole body all the way to the floor. It should pass through your center of gravity. It should line up with the ear lobe, with the center of the tip of the shoulder, with the hip joint, behind the patella (kneecap), and midway between the heel and the arch of the foot.

2. From the back (posterior) view, the plumb line should fall through the center of the skull, following the line of the spine and the hips (between the cheeks of the buttocks) down to the floor. The lower limbs should be spaced equidistant on either side of the line, and the knees and heels should line up directly below the hips. The knees, pelvis, and shoulders should be parallel to the floor.

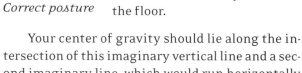

*Figure 22. Correct posture*

Your center of gravity should lie along the intersection of this imaginary vertical line and a second imaginary line, which would run horizontally in the area between your hips and your lower ribs.

## THE TRIPOD POSITION

To achieve overall balance of the body in a standing position, you should make sure that the feet evenly support the body when they are placed directly under the hip joints. The body's weight should be evenly distributed over three points that form a triangle on each foot:

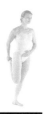

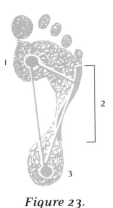

*Figure 23.
The tripod
position*

1. the ball of the big toe

2. the outside edge of the foot

3. the center of the heel

There should be no pressure forward on the toes or backward on the heels. By placing an equal pressure on the outside edge of the foot, you may feel as if you are creating an arch where the arch should be. Try to maintain this tripod position whenever standing.

## POSTURAL ASSESSMENT

Correct posture may be determined either by visual means or by actual measurement, which is useful when the eye cannot detect slight misalignments. The following are two main areas of the body where a person's posture can deviate from the norm:

1. The lower limbs: the feet, tibia/fibula, and femur.

2. The pelvis and torso: the pelvis, and the lumbar, thoracic, and cervical sections of the spine and rib cage.

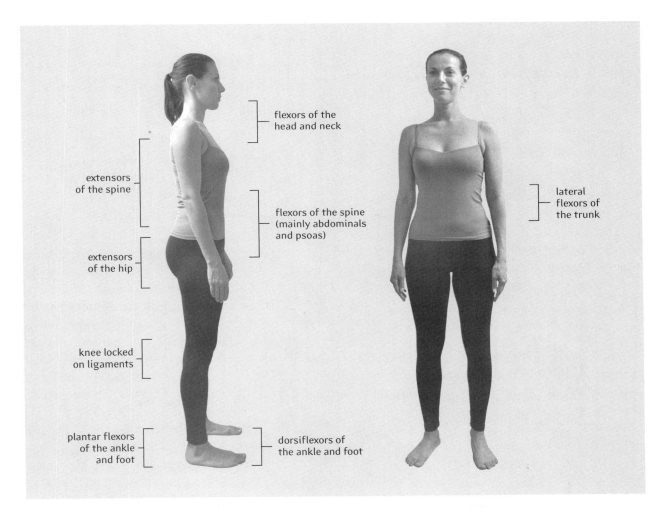

*Figure 24. The main muscle groups that control posture in a standing position*

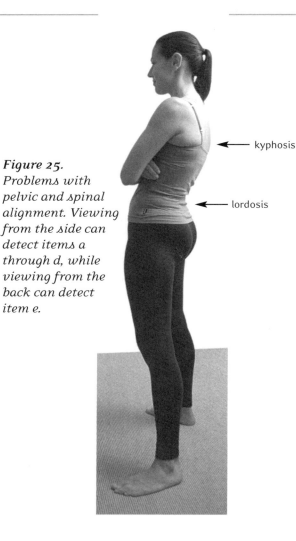

*Figure 25.
Problems with
pelvic and spinal
alignment. Viewing
from the side can
detect items a
through d, while
viewing from the
back can detect
item e.*

kyphosis

lordosis

Positions a, c, and d can be detected from a front view, and position b from a side view. Bad posture in the pelvis and torso can result from the following:

2. Problems with pelvic and spinal alignment (see Figure 25).

    a)  Anterior (forward) or posterior (backward) tilt of the pelvis

    b)  Lumbar lordosis (see "Anatomical Terms" in Chapter 2)

    c)  Kyphosis

    d)  Cervical lordosis

    e)  Scoliosis

3. Actions of the scapulae (shoulder blades) and shoulder

    a)  Elevation: hunched shoulders

    b)  Depression: pushed-down shoulders

    c)  Adduction: shoulders squeezed together

    d)  Abduction: winged shoulder blades

    e)  Forward rotation of the shoulders

## BAD POSTURE AND LOWER-BACK PAIN

The following is a common example of how bad posture can affect the lower back. Stand with your hands on your hips. This simple, seemingly innocent movement has no fewer than four detrimental effects on the body.

You will notice that the hands are usually placed with the fingers on the front of the hips and the thumbs hooked at the top of the hipbones at the back. Most people adopt this stance, especially if they have lower-back pain. Others may adopt the "preg-

Bad posture in the lower limbs can result from conditions such as the following:

1. Foot pronation (rolling inward) or supination (rolling outward), inversion (pointing inward) or eversion (pointing outward)

    a)  Knock-knees (genu valgum) and bow legs (genu varum)

    b)  Hyperextended or hyperflexed knees

    c)  Differences in leg length

    d)  Tibial torsion (when the feet are parallel and the knees roll in)

*Figure 26. Pregnancy stance*

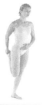

nancy" stance by placing the hands in the small of the back and pushing forward, creating a large arch in the lower back. In the long term, both stances, especially the pregnancy stance, cause the following in most individuals:

The pelvis tilts forward, leading to

1. Arching of the lower back, which causes these muscles to become shorter and tighter.

2. Shortening of the thigh muscles, which draws the pelvis farther forward, "locking" the hips. This is commonly seen in men with beer guts who are unable to tilt the pelvis backward.

3. Loosening and stretching of the lower abdominals.

4. Hunching of the shoulders, leading to tighter neck and chest muscles and looser muscles in the upper back.

## MUSCLE IMBALANCES

Muscles that overwork or strain on a frequent basis can cause an imbalance of the skeletal structure. It is commonly assumed that overworked muscles need stretching and underworked muscles require strengthening for the body to be in a position of balance or equilibrium. Postural defects that can be corrected are those that are created by weak or overstrong muscles.

The hip flexors (see Figures 27 and 28) have an enormous effect on the body's structure, especially its posture. The psoas major (also called *iliopsoas*) and iliacus, if overstrong, tend to lift or lurch the body from a flat (supine) position to sitting upright. In order to roll the spine into an upright position, these hip flexors need to be controlled by producing more mid- and lower-abdominal control.

Another group of hip flexors is the quadriceps or thigh muscles. There are four major groups of muscles in the thigh. (*Quad* is Latin for "four.") They attach from the top of the hip and femur to the patella (kneecap) and quadriceps tendon at the

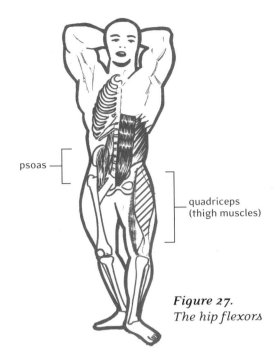

psoas

quadriceps (thigh muscles)

*Figure 27.*
*The hip flexors*

knee. Because they are the largest group of muscles in the body, they tend to do a great deal of work without any conscious effort involved. From when we are babies, with our legs in the air, to the time we crawl, to the time we stand erect to walk, run, or jump, the thigh muscles are continuously engaged.

Continually exposing these muscles to overexertion without opposite relief, such as stretching, can cause problems that include back pain as we grow into adulthood. When the muscles of the upper thigh are overstrong they tend to tilt the pelvis in an anterior (forward) position. This, in turn, tends to create a small arch in the lower back, lengthening the lower abdominals and causing the iliopsoas hip flexors to also shorten and accentuate the arch in the small of the back. Although the mid- and upper abdominals may appear flat, they may not be working hard enough to counter the strength of the hip flexors that pull the spine forward. This imbalance can cause considerable back pain. In general, we can equate back pain to a lack of muscle strength in a corresponding section of the abdominal area—for example, a tight lower back generally corresponds to weak lower abdominals (below the navel).

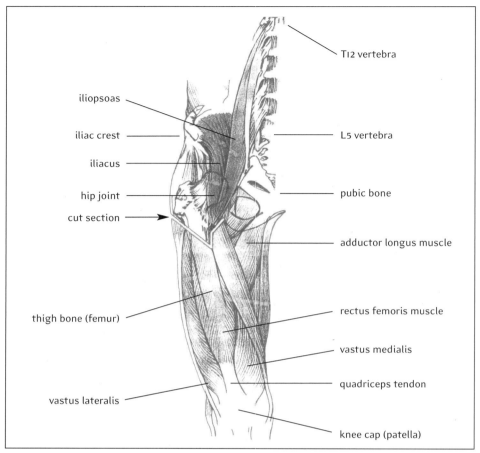

T12 vertebra

iliopsoas

iliac crest

L5 vertebra

iliacus

hip joint

pubic bone

cut section

adductor longus muscle

thigh bone (femur)

rectus femoris muscle

vastus medialis

quadriceps tendon

vastus lateralis

knee cap (patella)

*Figure 28. Front view—hip flexors (detail)*

As described above, a tightening of the thigh muscles can lead to an arching of the lower back. As this continues, the lower back and psoas muscles also become contracted, causing the psoas to draw the lumbar vertebrae forward. This creates stress on the spinal column and on the discs. This pressure, caused by a combination of tight back, psoas, and thigh muscles, can exert enough pressure on the spine to squeeze nerves between the disc and the vertebra, resulting in sciatic pain.

From this common example, we can recognize that muscles work in conjunction with each other. A chain reaction can occur when misalignment of muscles in one part of the body causes the need for a compensation in another part, farther up or down the line. In the above example, a further compensation for the hyperextension in the lower back (lumbar vertebrae) might result in a tendency to sway back at the knees.

## IDENTIFYING AND AVOIDING PAIN

Injuries occur even in people who are fit or who think they are fit. When an injury occurs, other muscles "seize" to "protect" the injured area. As a result, some of the muscles exert themselves more than usual. As they become stronger they tend to pull the body further out of alignment. So, once the original injury has been resolved, another problem has been created that requires correcting. Another common result of the body's overcompensation following an injury is wastage (atrophy) of muscles that fail to get used as often as they should. These muscles then need to be strengthened to bring the body back into balance. Although the person thinks he is healed, he may still be in pain because of increased pressure on the limbs or joints from other muscles that have been automatically recruited to keep the structure functioning as nor-

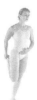

## JOANNE T.

*Joanne T., a sixteen-year-old female with a previous history of ballet and, more recently, gymnastics, saw her practitioner for mild but increasing lower-back pain. Her physique was that of a fit young girl with no postural deviations and flat abdominals. Upon examination by X ray and CAT scans, it was discovered that she had a mild posterior disc bulge at L4–5. The pain gradually became worse, with no alleviation of the symptoms from various forms of treatment. Her movements were akin to that of a fifty-year-old with severe back pain.*

*When Joanne T. came to the studio, it was discovered that her hip flexors were doing all the work and she had only minimal abdominal strength. Manual pressure was applied to the lower abdominals at the psoas level, and lower-limb activity was undertaken. These actions reduced her pain levels. Lower-abdominal work, especially focusing on the B-Line Core, was initiated. Joanne T.'s condition improved approximately 10 percent over four months. After twelve months of treatment in a studio situation, using equipment, her condition improved 80 percent. She now experiences only occasional setbacks in her progress.*

mally as possible. During exercise, you should never feel any pressure, strain, or pain in the following three areas:

1. The back

2. The neck

3. Any of the other joints

(Although the neck and back are joints, I have itemized them separately here for easier identification by those new to discovering their bodies through movement.)

If certain movements cause you pain in any of these three bodily areas, before beginning or con-

tinuing an exercise or sports program you should first take appropriate action to determine what causes the pain, and then employ clinical efforts (treatment, scans, etc.) to alleviate the problem. If the pain persists, before beginning or restarting an exercise program it is essential to take the following steps:

1. Identify the area of pain: muscle, joint, tissue, or bone.

2. Assess the level of pain during specific movements. (For instance, is pain present only when certain activities takes place?)

3. Determine the amount of restriction of the painful area.

4. Determine whether the area has suffered a previous injury or trauma.

5. Establish whether scar tissue is present that would further restrict the full range of motion.

Let's look in more detail at each of these specific types of pain.

### Joint Strains

Joint strains are fairly common and can be corrected quite easily in the early stages. If you experience any strain in any joint when exercising, it is important to do the following:

1. If the affected joint is a "ball and socket" or rotating joint (shoulder/hip), reduce the rotation of the joint (if externally or internally rotated at the joint).

2. If the strain persists, reduce the range of movement of the joint.

3. If the affected joint is a hinge joint (knee/elbow), reduce the extension or flexion at the hinge.

4. If the affected joint is a rotating joint, instead of extending (straightening) or locking the nearest hinge joint, introduce a slight bending, or flexion, of the hinge joint during your movements to better

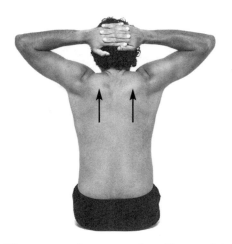

*Figure 29a. Incorrect shoulder position that causes neck strain*

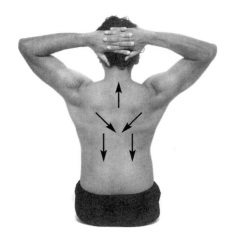

*Figure 29b. Correct shoulder position that creates perfect posture and reduces neck strain*

engage the muscle between the rotating joint and the hinge joint. For example, see the easier variation of Exercise 22 that calls for keeping the knee bent and placing the hand on the knee (Knee Stirs).

### Neck Strain

Neck strain usually occurs during exercise because the head is being held up off the ground continuously or because the movement of the head is causing a strain. When a person is in a supine position (lying on his or her back) doing an exercise that calls for lifting the head, it is not the fact that the head is lifted that causes most neck strain; it is the *distance* the head is moved that creates the most strain.

When exercising in a supine position, neck strain can in most cases be alleviated by following these steps:

1. Draw the ribs closer to the hips in a horizontal plane.

2. Draw the shoulder blades toward the tailbone.

3. Support the head with your hands or with a cushion (but make sure the cushion isn't too large, to prevent the head from being raised too high).

### Alleviating Lower-Back Strain by Decompressing the Spine

Lower-back strain during exercising is generally caused by the back arching or hyperextending. Try the following to alleviate lower-back strain:

1. When exercising in a supine position (lying on your back), lengthen the back by imprinting the spine onto the floor. Do this by curling the pelvis up, lightly grasping your buttocks with your hands, and then pressing the hips away from the ribs and towards the feet as you imprint the spine onto the floor. Now engage the B-Line Core. (For more detail about imprinting the spine from a sitting position, see page 53.) We will refer to this in the exercise descriptions as "decompressing the spine" or as the Stable Spine position. Now, remaining in this position, imagine two coins—one placed under your lumbar spine (at navel level), and the other placed under your sacrum (located where the spine meets the tailbone, just below the lumbar spine). We will refer to these throughout the book as either the "lumbar coin" or the "sacrum coin." When the knees are bent or the legs are in the air, imagine pressing the two coins into the floor using equal pressure.

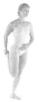

*Figure 30.* The stretch scale

| No stretch | mild stretch | | strong stretch | | stretch pain | "pain" pain (avoid!) |
|---|---|---|---|---|---|---|
| 0 . . . . . . . . . . . . . . 1 . . . 2 . . . 3 . . . 4 . . . 5 . . . . . . . . . . 6 . . . . . . 7 . . . . . 8 . . . . . . . . . . . . . . . . . . . 9 . . . . . . . . . . . . 10 | | | | | | |
| SAFE | | | WORK | | DANGER | |

2. If, after following step 1, your back is still arched, first do some thigh stretches (see Exercises 11-13) to mobilize the hip joints. This may alleviate the problem almost immediately for a short period of time, but the stretches must be continued on a regular basis to maintain the improvement.

3. Tilt the pelvis under slightly (posterior tilt) to correct the arch. If you're lying down, do not lift the hips off the floor (i.e., continue pressing the coin beneath the sacrum).

4. If you are lying down with the knees bent and the back is still arched, then draw the knees to the chest.

5. If you are standing, draw the rib cage to the imaginary wall without rounding the shoulders or bending the knees.

## LISTENING TO YOUR BODY FOR GREATER RESULTS: THE STRETCH SCALE AND THE WORK SCALE

When following an exercise or stretching routine, it is important to listen to what your body is telling you. The myth of "No pain, no gain" is old-fashioned and dangerous. The pain you feel could actually be tears in the microfibers of the muscle itself. At the same time, however, a certain amount of discomfort will occur during training, even after proper warming up. In order to challenge ourselves to become better at any physical activity, a certain discomfort level is acceptable. The real question is up to what level is discomfort acceptable? A very mild, tolerable, uncomfortable, but not burning sensation in the working muscles is okay.

In any case, if the pain is sudden, sharp, uncomfortable, or acute, our body is telling us that we must cease that activity.

In addition, if you have not worked out for some time and decide to engage in even a mild circuit class, then you are likely to feel a certain amount of soreness the next day. It is best to do a correctly executed stretching routine before the start of a class or to participate in a mild stretch class the next day to alleviate most aches and pains from the previous day.

Stretching the muscles should be performed gradually. Continual working and stretching through pain is not an intelligent approach to good body maintenance. The muscles need time to repair themselves before further exertion is applied to them. In the long term, overdoing it could lead to those niggling, recurring complaints that can haunt you for years. If you have this problem, consult a trained, exercise-oriented health-care professional or a qualified Pilates instructor.

While exercising, it may be useful to adopt the following stretch scale guideline to assess the intensity of your stretching activities. Note: If you experience any unusual twinges or momentarily sharp pain, reduce the exercise or stretch to a level that is comfortable.

### The Stretch Scale from 0 to 10

- 0-6 = No Progress: In this range you may feel a mild stretch, but no progress is made.

- 6.05-8.95 = Progress: Between levels 6 and 8.95, you will experience a strong muscular stretch which produces results. You know you are really doing some work. You are being challenged at this level. If you are

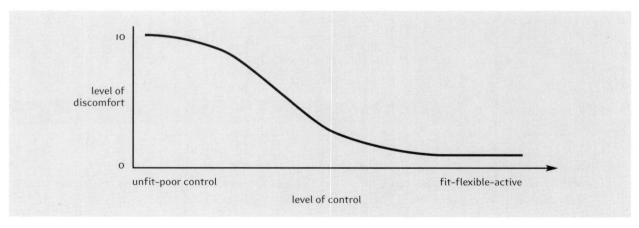

*Figure 31. The activity chart. The less active we are, the more discomfort we feel, whereas the more active we are, the less likely we are to experience long-lasting aches and pains.*

only at level 6, gradually increase your intensity toward 8.95.

- **9 = Borderline Pain:** When approaching level 9, the feel of the stretch or movement changes from one of comfort to one of discomfort or mild pain. Only the quadriceps stretch should be done at this level. In this zone, damage may occur in the form of microfiber tears of the muscle. It is better to back off from this level of exercise rather than risk forcing the muscles and possibly causing injury.

- **10 = "Pain" Pain:** Level 10 is unbearable pain and should always be avoided.

Only very experienced athletes who understand their bodies through many years of training (and, usually, many injuries) would experience any benefit from working in what to most of us is the danger zone (levels 9 and 10). Athletes of this caliber have a heightened body awareness, not only because of the stringent demands they make on their bodies but also as a result of the mental discipline required to attain the best results.

The work scale is a guideline to assess muscular effort. Like the stretch scale, the work scale also relies on a scale of 0 to 10. When you're exercising,

ask yourself how intensely you're working. Interpret your response based on the following scale:

### The Work Scale from 0 to 10

**0-6 = NO PROGRESS:** No work at all.

**6.05-8.95 = PROGRESS:** At this level the exercise is a challenge. If you continuously work within this comfortable level, you will always see results.

**9 = STRUGGLE:** Exercise at this level is uncomfortable; your muscles start to shake.

**10 = COLLAPSE:** You cannot proceed any further. Remember: it is far better to do four repetitions correctly than ten incorrectly!

*The stretch scale always dictates.* By this I mean if your exertion level registers an 8 on the stretch scale but only a 3 on the work scale, for that particular exercise, the 8 level is to be observed. In other words, do not push yourself further along the work scale to attain its challenge range (6.05-8.95). Doing so will only push you further on the stretch scale into the danger zone. As you continue doing the routines on a regular basis, your position on the stretch scale for the exercise in question may ease back to 6 or so. In this case, your effort on the work scale can then be increased to 4 or 5, and so on.

## BODY POSITIONING FOR BETTER EXERCISING

**B**efore beginning any exercise, it is essential to assume the correct posture or position in order to connect or engage the appropriate muscle groups. When you assume the correct posture, your energy is focused on the muscles involved to work and avoids being wasted on other areas of the body or on unnecessary movements.

This is especially true when beginning an exercise that is totally new to your body. New exercise programs generally require concentration and control to which the body may never have been subjected. For instance, suppose a triathlete attempts a yoga class for the first time. The new positions require a great deal of thought and focus. Muscles are being subjected to movements that are new to them, and forcing the movements can cause injury, especially if the positions are held for some time. It is always important to keep in mind that any new bodily routine must be approached with caution.

Because triathletes are quite fit compared to the general population, they also approach physical challenges more readily and sometimes throw themselves into new regimes with the mental attitude that their bodies can endure any new venture. The muscles, however, have memorized only certain movements as a result of countless hours of repeating those movements over many years. Once the body and mind have approached a routine in a certain manner, it is difficult to change that pattern without creating changes to the results. These changes may initially be adverse—such as slower times or shorter jumping distances—until the muscles accept their new regime as the basis upon which to progress. Accordingly, if an athlete undertakes Pilates he or she will initially see negative results until the body "tunes" itself to the new regime. Then the results will be seen in faster times, greater distances, and the like. It is essential, therefore, for athletes to work with an appropriately trained Pilates instructor—one who has great knowledge and specific training in athletic movement, rather than a ballet-trained Pilates instructor, who may have less refined experience in athletics.

Our bodies will invariably take the easy way out. They will perform movements that require the least effort and concentration. When we are not focused, *our bodies will cheat on us!* To illustrate this, lie on your back with your arms extended toward the ceiling above your chest. This may be done with or without hand weights. If you use weights, hold them directly above the chest, in line with the shoulders. Slowly open the arms out to the sides away from the body, and then close them again above your chest. Repeat the movement half a dozen times. Notice that as you do more repetitions, the arms slowly start to move above the face when in the air, and in line with the head when open to the floor. This has the effect of gradually raising the shoulders and engaging the neck muscle. Imagine the effect when the exercise is repeated hundreds of times!

To work specific muscle groups requires concentration and effort. To execute a near-perfect movement until the muscle forms an engram (subconscious pattern) that will make the movement automatic requires a "pattern" of sorts for muscular development. To accomplish this, you need to establish a focused routine. Then any new movements, such as an attempt at yoga when you've previously been a triathlete, can be approached safely. You can perform your own "self-check" as to the requirements, benefits, limits, and dangers to which your body will be exposed.

## THE EXERCISE FORMULA

**I** have developed a formula that will help you perform any exercise to the best of your physical ability, no matter what your level of fitness. The formula has been designed to help you make each exercise precise and thus help you gain the most benefit from each movement or series of movements.

At first, it may seem difficult to follow all the points of the formula at the same time. However, by systematically covering each point sequentially and mastering that principle before undertaking the next, you can perfect the exercise and develop great technique. A gradual, step-by-step approach to a new routine will establish a solid foundation for developing greater speed, range, or control in the movement.

The formula is as follows:

1. Posture/Alignment/Position

2. Back

3. Breathing

4. Exercise

5. Elongation

6. Questions

It has been found that if the formula is adhered to, it is almost impossible to perform a routine incorrectly, or for an instructor to teach an incorrect movement to a client.

Let's look at each of these six points in turn.

### 1. Posture/Alignment/Position

When beginning an exercise, it is important to first establish the correct position or alignment for the exercise. If it is not correct from the start, the movement will probably be sloppy and less effective. This is especially important for rehabilitation exercise programs. Establishing and maintaining the correct position of a limb, the pelvis, or the torso is crucial to the final outcome. A difference of even one centimeter in the position of a body part can mean a difference of 10 to 50 percent in the effectiveness of the exercise. Imagine a gymnast on the parallel bars or on the beam who moves one centimeter off her projected alignment. She may lose control or balance or fall off the apparatus. Or if a tennis player misses the "sweet spot" on his racquet more times than his opponent does, it could mean the difference between winning and losing, between perfection and "close enough is good enough." The same is true in developing the type of body you really want.

Training the brain to search for these small differences requires assistance. A mirror can help you identify major differences in position and alignment.

The following are some questions to ask yourself when practicing this principle of the formula. Keep in mind that the list is not exhaustive.

1. Are the hips square?

2. Is the leg in line with the shoulder?

3. Is the torso upright?

4. Is the foot flexed (or pointed)?

5. Are the shoulders level?

6. Is the back straight?

7. Is the stomach flat?

8. Is the neck elongated?

9. Are the shoulders relaxed?

### 2. Back

Ensure that the back is in the required position for the start of the exercise. Generally, when you are lying supine with the knees bent and the feet flat on the floor, the back should be in the Stable Spine position with the B-Line Core engaged. Now also engage the pelvic floor as previously described.

This may be one of the few times many of us actually feel our lower abdominals contracting! Continually maintaining the B-Line Core helps to strengthen this group of abdominal muscles. Strength in the lower abdominals greatly assists in the relief of lower-back pain and in the ability to mobilize the pelvis.

Control of the rib cage also provides stability for the spine (see the section that follows, on breathing). When we are upright, is the back straight or is there a lean to one side? Is the lower back arched or the upper back too rounded? Is the head tilted forward or backward? All these problems can be corrected to a certain extent by realignment and reeducation of the muscles. If the problem is more structural, as in some cases of osteoporosis, the spine and back should be aligned as well as possible, without causing any discomfort.

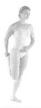

### 3. Breathing

We discussed breathing in Chapter 2. However, the proper method of breathing is important and cannot be stressed too often. When performing challenging small movements, many people hold their breath. As I mentioned earlier, it is important to avoid holding the breath while exercising. If you hold your breath while performing a movement, you will strain your body.

It is generally accepted that when exercising one should breathe out on the effort. In the style of Pilates outlined in this book sometimes the breathing is *reverse* to this principle. That's because in some cases breathing *in* on the effort provides more support for the back. For example, imagine you are lying on your back on a low bench, lifting a heavy weight to work the triceps. To perform this movement, you bend the elbows of both arms, lowering the weight above the head toward the floor, and then straighten the elbows to return the arms to the vertical position. There are several problems with how this action is typically performed.

This movement is usually done with the feet on the ground, creating an arch in the lower back before the exercise has even begun. This by itself can cause stress and tightening in the lower-back muscles. When you lower the weight toward the floor, the back then arches even further as the pectorals almost lock at a certain point. There is limited mobility at the shoulder joint. You usually take a short breath in as the arms lower toward the floor and a heavy breath out as you raise the arms back to the starting position. All of this results in a great deal of strain on the entire torso.

To control the exercise and to focus the work on the targeted muscle group, other areas of stress and strain should be eliminated as much as possible. The breathing is usually one such stress point. Breathing plays an important role in helping the body to cope with stress, whether mental or physical. If you were to perform the same exercise with calmer breathing, a flatter back, and less facial expression, the exercise would look very easy. You might also need to lighten the weight to gain

more control, because the different method of breathing would change your muscles' ability to perform the movement as they were used to doing previously.

Often, when people are instructed to breathe during an exercise, they are told something like this: "Lift your leg and breathe out." They may interpret this to mean that they are to move the limb and then, at the completion of the movement, to breathe out. Instead, as discussed in Chapter 2, the breathing instruction should ideally be phrased something as follows: "Breathe in (or out) to...." Breathe for the duration of the movement to reduce stresses and strains, thereby avoiding injury. Breathe calmly in through the nose, and ocean breathe out through the mouth.

As you become accustomed to breathing in the manner appropriate for the movement, you can do faster repetitions, still breathing *in* normally for two, three, or four repetitions and *out* for the next two, three, or four reps. Controlled, calm breathing can enhance physical performance.

### 4. Exercise

When you get to this step, you are performing the exercise as perfectly as possible. If you are unable to perfect the exercise with the correct breathing in the first half dozen movements, do not despair. Practice the exercise with whatever breathing feels comfortable. Get the body to move and to understand what is required of it. As doing this becomes more feasible and familiar, then adjust the breathing to the correct requirements.

Even when performing advanced exercises, return to the basic versions every so often. You will find that they, too, can still challenge you as you learn to apply more focus and connection to the simpler movements.

### 5. Elongation

When moving the limbs or any other part of the body, you can gain a greater feeling of working all the muscles, especially the unused, smaller ones, by lengthening through the movement. For example, when standing or lying on your back, engage the B-Line Core and decompress the spine (drawing ribs away from hips), while at the same time pressing the shoulder blades toward the tailbone. This action requires greater abdominal contraction and helps to keep the spine longer and more flexible, as well as alleviating pressure on the vertebrae and discs.

When working on lengthening the arms or legs, keep the knee and elbow joints slightly unlocked (avoid hyperextension). Locking them can cause stress on those joints. If these joints are hyperextended, then the bones are merely being locked together and the muscles will strain rather than work. You should also avoid too much of a bend (hyperflexion), which will prevent the muscle from lengthening and will restrict mobility of the limb from the socket. With the joint unlocked it is still possible to lengthen out of the socket (without moving the hip or shoulder) to attain the mobility required.

Continual lengthening of the muscle group being worked can result in several distinct benefits, including the following:

- Leaner muscles, less bulk

- Reduced stress on the joint

- Increased awareness of specific, isolated muscle movement

- Increased mobility of the joint

- Reduced "clicking" of the joint

The muscle group you wish to lengthen should be stable and injury-free. Lengthening of injured muscles can place more load on the fibers and lead to further problems.

In many exercise routines, especially those involving heavy weights, it is common for the limb to be unable to move through its full range. The body keeps the limb from extending in order to reduce the amount of stress on the joint. However, failing to extend the muscle through its full range has the effect of shortening the muscle. During biceps curls, for example, when lifting a heavy weight, the

arm is rarely extended close to its full length. The upper body is usually also curled forward in order to prepare it to take the strain of the next lift. The movement of the weight touching the thigh gives the illusion that the arm has performed close to a full extension.

If the exercise were performed correctly—that is, through the full range—with the same amount of effort, the weight would need to be reduced, because the biceps muscle fiber is weaker when it is almost fully extended. Once greater strength is achieved in the extended position, then an increased weight can be safely applied.

Similarly, during an abdominal curl, if the knees are bent at an acute angle at the knee joint (heels too close to the bottom), there is less chance of achieving length in the abdominals. The forward contraction has the effect of squashing the abdominals and causing the front of the thighs to grip. This makes the abs bulge upward rather than scoop. The exercise then becomes strained and ineffective.

With the knee joint at a right angle (feet farther away from the bottom), performance can improve, with increased effect on the muscle worked, as long as the abdominals are scooped in. With the knee joint at greater than a right angle (obtuse angle), the hip flexors are more elongated, and, if the Stable Spine and B-Line Core are engaged, the exercise is more challenging. If the pull of the hip flexors is further reduced, the abdominals will work more effectively (see Exercise 25 with cushion under the knees).

Strength in length would be the epitome of muscle tone for almost every athlete. Female classical ballet dancers find that they are extremely flexible but not strong enough in their extreme ranges of movement. To them this is a weakness. But however desirable the strength factor is to them, most ballet dancers would not be caught dead in a weight-training gym, for fear their muscles would become too bulky!

On the other hand, triathletes would welcome more flexibility without compromising their strength. But most of them would never be caught dead in a ballet class! The Pilates techniques out-

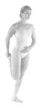

lined in this book can cater to both groups. Dancers can, with the correct use of weights, gain greater strength without fear of bulking their muscles. Triathletes can improve their flexibility without compromising their strength or speed. In fact, both could benefit from one common factor: the reduced risk of injury.

Elongation through the full range of movement and during all repetitions requires concentration and effort. As the muscle tires, the first thing to happen is the reduction in the lengthening of the muscle. This happens because the muscle can work more easily in a contracted position. When you find that you cannot maintain your muscle elongation, stop the exercise. Continue only when you are able to maintain an elongated line.

### 6. Questions

This is the most important part of the Exercise Formula as it requires feedback. Using the feedback we "rearrange" the exercise, if necessary, to produce greater results.

Once the preceding five principles of the formula have been systematically performed, the final and most important part of the equation remains. Even when you have mentally assessed and corrected each movement, there might still be room for improvement in your technique. There are several ways to assess your performance. Asking yourself the following question can help you correct the movement by returning to the formula:

*Where do you feel the exercise working, and at what level on the work scale or stretch scale (whichever applies to the exercise)?*

You should feel the exercise working *only* in the muscle groups intended for that movement. There are many areas where things can go wrong. The rule is, if it feels uncomfortable or hurts, don't do it!

Common sense should dictate your actions at all times. Some of the most important areas to focus on are listed in the following section. It is by no means an exhaustive list, but, as a guide, it can introduce an understanding of correct and safe muscle movement. Following it can give you a greater sense of awareness of the moving body and encourage you to listen to your body when it talks to you.

## BODY AWARENESS AND POSTURE

Getting to know your body is an important start to your Pilates program or any other exercise program. As people develop physically, they also develop physical habits. Some of these may have taken years to develop, such as lifting objects in a certain way. Whatever the reason, when performing any task our bodies prefer to move along the path of least resistance. That path is accommodated by our subconscious. It is stored in our memory banks for future reference when we make the same, or similar, movements. Our bodies will automatically want to cheat on us when we perform many of life's everyday movements.

Many of these movements may be incorrect, such as walking with the arches of our feet dropped inward (pronated). This may explain why some people get headaches and others get lower-back pain. However, most of us are unaware that such a movement could be the cause of our symptoms. Understanding and correcting the body's smallest imbalances and incorrect positions can eliminate many of the minor, or major, aches and pains we become so accustomed to living with.

By becoming more aware of your body, and of the space within which it moves, you can gain greater understanding of your physical being. Mentally identifying and feeling individual parts of your body without having to move those parts may be difficult at first. However, when you achieve this, you can more easily understand how to move correctly. The result is that your physical and mental reflexes become more heightened, you can judge distances better, control the amount of effort you apply to physical tasks, and even relieve physical stress and mental anxiety.

Understanding your body also means listening to it when it reacts adversely to situations. It means not pushing it when you think you can perform a task but you realize that physically you have even slight doubts. As you develop your body with this program, you will begin to realize that without correct mental focus, your movements become sloppy and ineffective. It is important to understand that when your body has performed several repetitions of a movement as correctly as possible, and the extra one is not up to standard, then you should not continue with the remaining repetitions. One perfectly executed movement is worth any number of sloppy ones!

Several key concepts are essential to the basic control of the exercises and the achievement of beneficial results. A few of them are listed below:

- When you think you have gone as far as you can, extend it!

- To be terrific, you have to be specific.

- Rotate from the rib cage.

- Draw the shoulder blades into the pocket (toward the tailbone).

- If it's out of alignment, align it.

- If a muscle is not working, make it work.

- The breathing makes the exercise.

- Breathing out more forcefully helps to activate the deepest layer of the abdominal muscles (the transversus abdominis, see Figure 36).

- Where the eyes go, the body follows.

- Work the muscle closest to the rotating joint or fulcrum.

## THE PERFECT TORSO POSTURE (PTP)

As was stated earlier in this chapter, when moving the limbs or any other part of the body, you can gain a greater sense of working all the muscles, especially the unused, smaller ones, by lengthening or elongating through the movement. To do this for the torso, and thereby achieve what I call the Perfect Torso Posture, follow the steps listed below when sitting or standing:

1. Engage the B-Line Core.

2. Keep the ribs lengthened away from the hips at the sides (lateral).

3. Press the shoulder blades toward the tailbone (which we shall call the "pocket").

4. Lengthen through the crown of the head, and drop the tailbone to the floor.

5. When in a supine position (lying on your back) with the knees bent or with the legs in the air rather than extended on the ground, decompress the spine by lengthening the hips away from the ribs.

## ESTABLISHING CORRECT POSTURE

### Foot Positions

Your posture starts from your feet!

The feet are an integral part of any exercise. Not to be regarded just as attachments at the end of our legs, the feet are continuously working. At no time should they be flopping around and left unattended.

When standing, imagine that each of your feet is like a tripod (see "The Tripod Position," earlier in this chapter). When you maintain this equal loading while moving the rest of the body, you will feel as if you were anchored to the floor. In this way, you can achieve a key element of good posture. Work the abdominals as described below, keeping the legs straight but not locked. Engage the Perfect Torso Posture.

In the pointed position (Figure 32a), the feet are pointed, with the joint between the big toe and the second toe in line with the center of the kneecap. This line of strength prevents the foot from ei-

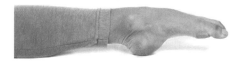

*Figure 32a. In the pointed position (plantar flexion)*

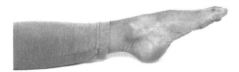

*Figure 32b. Softly pointed feet*

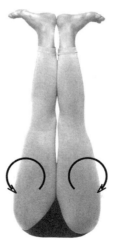

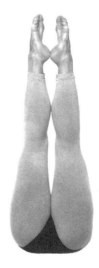

*Figure 35a.*
*Legs extended, feet*
*flexed and turned out*

*Figure 35b.*
*Legs extended, feet*
*pointed and turned out*

ther inversion (turning in, see Figure 33) or eversion (turning out). The stretch should be felt on the top of the foot, and you should feel a lengthening sensation rather than a cramped pointing of the toes. Attempting to overstretch through the toes can result in a cramping of the arches of the feet. If this occurs, softly point the feet (Figure 32b).

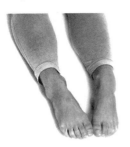

*Figure 33.*
*Inverted (sickle) feet*

To achieve the flexed position, or dorsiflexion (Figure 34), press through the heels as far as possible. This should draw the toes toward your knees without curling them back. If the toes do tend to curl back, draw the balls of your feet toward you. This may take some practice. If, when you flex the feet, the calves feel excessively tight, stretch them before continuing with the rest of the program.

In Figures 35a and 35b, the feet are shown both flexed and turned out, and pointed and turned out. When turning out, imagine the muscles of the inner thigh doing the work, rather than forcing the rotation from the knees or the feet.

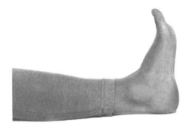

*Figure 34. Flexed position (dorsiflexion)*

### Toning

Most women would like to tone the following muscle areas:

- The backs of the arms
- The section of the abdominals below the navel
- The buttocks
- The outside of the hips
- The backs of the thighs

Most men are principally interested in toning the entire abdominal area.

If we could keep the muscles toned, fatty deposits would have less chance of accumulating in these areas. For example, how often do we find fatty deposits on the front of the thighs? Because we are continuously walking, climbing stairs, jogging, or running, the quadriceps muscles rarely have a chance to rest. We do not have to worry about toning this group.

By contrast, the buttocks are not typically held firm in our normal, daily routines. Hence, the muscles there become slack and require extra work to reshape them to the desired size or shape. Squeezing the buttocks tightly as though they were gripping a $100 bill is not essential to maintaining good tone and may ultimately produce more bulk in the buttocks as well as tension in the lower back. When standing, it is preferable to keep the buttocks pinched lightly, as if you were holding a $1 bill between your "cheeks." The following subsection discusses another method for toning this part of the body.

### The Bent-Knee Walk

To reduce back stress and tone the buttocks, walk with a tiny bend in the knees when the front foot hits the ground. Doing this may take some getting used to and feel unnatural at first, so let me break down the action for you.

First, walk normally, and as you're doing so place your hands on your buttocks. Are they firm or flabbing? Now walk with a tiny bend in the front knee, as if you were creeping up on someone (that is, land heel first and then roll forward to the toe, as usual). Use your hands to feel the difference in the muscle connection in the buttocks. You bend your knees when you walk downstairs, so why not do so when you're walking on a horizontal surface? Walking this way will:

- reduce stress in the knee joint because the action uses the knee as a spring rather than as a locked joint;

- reduce stress in the lower back by preventing the whole leg from jamming into the hip socket;

- eliminate jarring in the spine.

After walking with bent knees for thirty or forty steps, return to your normal gait and notice the difference. Do you feel the jarring and the banging of your heel on the ground?

### The Center (Abdominals)

Recall from the discussion of the eight Pilates principles (see Chapter 2) that the body's center is defined as the area between the ribs and the hips, which includes the front, back, and side muscles. It includes the four abdominal groups (see Figure 36) as well as the muscles of the back (quadratus lumborum) and on either side of the spine (erector spinae muscles). The abdominals provide support for the back in its function of keeping the body erect. They also assist in the rotation of the torso.

How they work to support the posture is easily illustrated: allow your stomach muscles to go slack. Notice what happens to your posture: You begin to slump. The shoulders move forward and down, the lower back arches, and the body becomes shorter. A slumping posture can lead to reduced breathing capacity as the lungs become squashed. Now sit upright on your sitz bones without arching the back. (When you sit as upright as possible without arching the back, can you feel the two bones in your bottom that you are sitting on? They are known as the "sitz bones.") Notice that at once your stomach pulls in toward your spine. The lower-back muscles also engage to straighten the

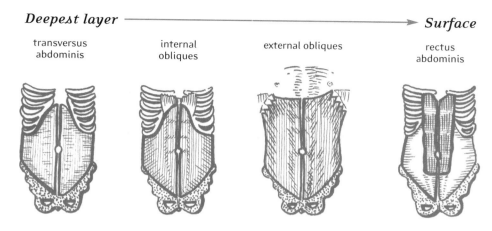

*Deepest layer* ——————————————————→ *Surface*

transversus abdominis     internal obliques     external obliques     rectus abdominis

*Figure 36. Abdominal muscles*

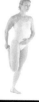

back. This has the effect not only of making you sit taller but also of supporting the back and lifting pressure off of it.

### Supine Position: Lying on Your Back

Place a mat on the floor and lie down on your back, feet extended and together and hands relaxed by your sides. You will observe that there is an arch in the lower back (neutral spine, Figure 37a). If this position is too uncomfortable, bend both legs very slightly. Place your hand in the space between your back and the floor, and engage the B-Line Core. Can you feel the abdominal muscles engaging? (Do not push your feet into the floor or tilt your pelvis up toward the ceiling.)

Remove your hand and continue to maintain the B-Line Core. Can you feel how much more deeply you are now working from the abdominal area? You may even feel as if the back itself is pressing to the floor (Stable Spine, Figure 37b). This is one method of identifying and feeling your "center." It is the area from which all controlled strength and flowing movement emanate.

Let's review how to engage the Stable Spine. First, decompress the spine, and then lengthen the hips away from the ribs. Now press the sacrum and lower lumbar sections of your back into the floor as though you're pressing down on two coins; do this without tilting the pelvis. This is the Stable Spine.

It is a common error to feel that if the back is not flat on the floor, then the back is not flat. The goal of the Stable Spine position is to keep the back supported while the spine is in a stable position, one in which the hips are neither tilted in a tuck nor extended to arch the back.

### The Neck

When lying on your back, do not allow the neck to arch, as doing so will tighten the neck muscles and jut the chin forward. Lengthen the crown of the head to stretch the neck muscles and to improve thoracic/cervical postural muscles. The eyes should be focused at an angle slightly forward of an imaginary vertical line from the eyes to the ceiling.

Tension in the neck (and shoulders) can lead to poor posture and severe headaches. Tight trapezius and cervical muscles make the chin jut forward and create an arch in the neck. To create positive muscle control, when sitting press the shoulder blades to the pocket and slowly draw the tip of the chin very slightly down toward the rib cage and slightly back toward the wall behind you, while lengthening the crown of the head to the ceiling (Figure 38b). Do not squash the chin to the chest. Can you feel the stretch in the back of the neck? This feeling may even extend down the upper back toward the shoulder blades.

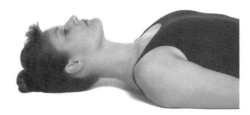

*Figure 38a. Do not allow the neck to arch*

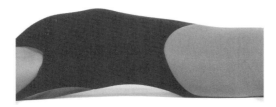

*Figure 37a. Neutral spine*

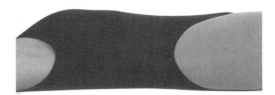

*Figure 37b. Stable spine*

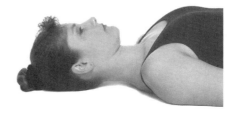

*Figure 38b. Lengthen the back of the neck*

## Sitting

When in a sitting position, most people have the tendency to slump (Figure 39a). Instead, when you're sitting, engage the Perfect Torso Posture. Imagine that your spine is similar to a rod. The rod is perfectly upright, perpendicular to the floor, running from the base of your spine through the crown of your head. Now imagine that your torso is sliding up the rod while your hips remain anchored to the ground, and engage the B-Line Core (Figure 39b. The body is straight and there is no arch in the back. If you had to sit with your legs straight in front of you, any arch in your back would immediately disappear. If you tried to create an arch in your back in this position you would undoubtedly strain your back muscles.

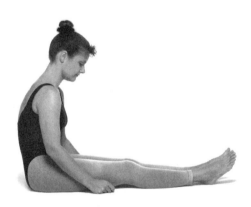

*Figure 39a. Incorrect sitting position*

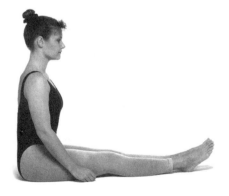

*Figure 39b. In a sitting position, perfectly upright*

## The Shoulders

Neck and shoulder tension is a common problem for most people, whether they exercise or not. This tension is caused by a tightening in the trapezius muscles. Often when we encounter a sudden shock or surprise, our arms, shoulders, and neck immediately tense in an almost defensive reaction. When we lift objects, even when we hold a baby on the hip, we hunch the shoulders. Then, when our friends give us a neck or shoulder rub, they comment on how these muscles are "as hard as rocks."

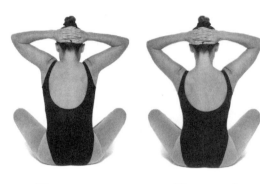

| Figure 40a. | Figure 40b. |
|---|---|
| *Incorrect* | *Correct* |

Neck and shoulder tension can be caused by situations as various as sitting in front of a typewriter or computer all day, or worrying about the results of an exam. Tension shortens the muscle group, as tension does with any muscles, which in turn hunches (and slightly rounds) the shoulders and arches the neck. To reverse this process, sit in an upright position with your hands behind your head and hunch your shoulders. Now, gently allow the shoulders to release by pressing the shoulder blades together and down toward the floor as hard as you can, while lengthening the crown of the head to the ceiling. (See Figures 40a and b.) This has the effect of opening the chest and allowing a slight release of the pectoral muscles that round the shoulders forward. It may even cause some discomfort between the shoulder blades as the muscles connect. Repeat this movement several times, and feel the tension release further each time.

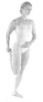

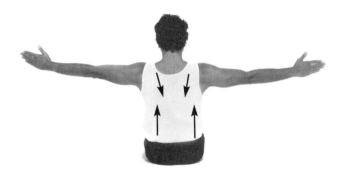

*Figure 41. Press shoulder blades to floor, lift ribs from hips*

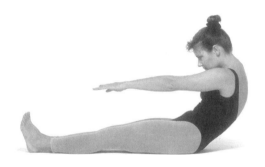

*Figure 42. Imprinting*

Another method of feeling the tension release is to place your hands on the top of your shoulders (right hand on right shoulder, left hand on left shoulder), with the elbows wide open. With your fingers, feel the tightness of the muscle here (the upper trapezius) as it remains in a contracted position. Now, keeping the fingers in place, simply draw your elbows toward each other in front of you, and feel the tension release from the muscle. It is better to have your elbows together than wide open.

For another method, sit with your arms extended away from the body at shoulder height, lengthening through your fingertips (Figure 41). Your neck and shoulders may already feel tense. Hunch them up as much as you can. Do you notice that the chin also tends to jut forward?

Now focus on the following:

1. Press the shoulder blades toward the pocket, with a deep sigh out.

2. Lengthen farther through the fingertips.

3. Grow as tall as you can out of your hips.

Repeat the movement by hunching only 10 percent as much as before. Now perform the release procedure above, and hold it for twenty seconds while breathing normally. Repeat four more times, and then rest your hands by your sides. Do you feel taller? More relaxed? Does your body feel lighter? Do you feel more relaxed mentally? By contracting the muscles opposite the ones that automatically create the tension, you can use positive muscle control to negate the effects of both physical and mental tension. (In this case, to counteract the pectoral muscles of the chest, which create rounded shoulders and a slumped posture, you're contracting the rhomboid muscles between the shoulder blades.)

### Imprinting and Peeling Off

Because the spine is a major focal point of movement for the rest of the body, it is important to keep it supple and strong. The movement of the spine when you get up off the floor or lie down should resemble that of leaving an imprint of the spine in soft sand. When you lower or raise the torso to or from the floor, each vertebra should be moved one at a time, without any sharp or jerky movements. Some analogies may help you to achieve this:

1. Imagine that the spine is like a string of pearls being lowered (or raised) one at a time.

2. Imagine that your spine is stuck to the perimeter of a wheel; as the wheel smoothly turns, so does each vertebra move one at a time, whether you're imprinting or peeling off the floor.

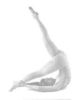

# 4

# Making Your Pilates Workout Effective and Safe

There are
only three things
in life that will
help us to live
longer: strength,
suppleness, and
a good sense of
humor.

— A. Menezes

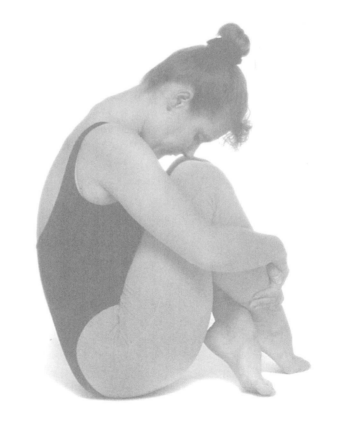

Although this book promotes isolation of muscles to attain a leaner, longer body with control and precision of movement, it is important to keep in mind that the body works as a whole. When you attempt to isolate a particular muscle for a stretch, other muscles may come into play. It is true that the toe bone is connected to the cheek bone via a complex arrangement of tissue, muscles, connecting joints, and mental perception.

## WARM-UP AND STRETCHING BEFORE YOUR WORKOUT

Stretching is an all-important part of warming up the muscles before any physical activity. It "wakes up" the muscles by providing an infusion of blood and nutrients into the open tissue. This makes the muscles more pliable and flexible, and the underlying joints able to move more freely.

Flexibility is defined as "the range of movement of a specific joint or group of joints influenced by the associated bones and bony structures and the physiological characteristics of the muscles, tendons, ligaments, and various other collagenous tissues surrounding the joint" (Arnheim, *Modern Principles of Athletic Training*. See References). Combining all of the principles we have discussed so far can lead to increased flexibility of the joints and better physical performance. Further means of achieving flexibility, such as specific muscle-stretching techniques, can also lead to greater results. I have devoted an entire section to flexibility and stretching, as this is extremely important in the prevention of injuries (see Chapter 5, "The Warm-Up").

Too much flexibility can lead to loss of muscular control, and too little can restrict movement. Both conditions can lead to injury. As an example of the former, classical ballet dancers are generally thought to be extremely flexible. However, many of them would like to have more strength in the extreme ranges of movement without compromising their flexibility or building bulk. At the other end of the spectrum, many triathletes feel they are too tight and would like to have more flexibility, and

thereby achieve better times, without compromising their strength.

There are two main types of stretches: dynamic (involving motion) and static (involving no motion).

The following sensible practices should be followed when performing stretches:

1. Stretch the muscle gradually.

2. If you feel any pain in the joints or elsewhere, reduce the pressure on the joint by following either suggestion below. After following these suggestions, if you still feel pain, do not continue.

   a) Reduce the angle at the joint. For example, when you do a seated hamstring stretch, if you feel more pain behind the knee joint than in the hamstring, bend the knee until you feel more of a hamstring stretch.

   b) Control the rotation of the joint. For example, if when you perform side splits (to stretch the adductors, or inner thigh muscles) you feel pressure in the knee joint, this may be because the femur (thigh bone) is rotating inward. Externally rotate the thigh until you feel only the adductor. To do this, depending on your level of flexibility, you may need to bring your legs slightly closer together.

3. Do not stretch injured or torn muscles.

4. If you have achieved maximum range of movement and still do not feel the stretch, continue the movement as a means of mobilizing the joint and loosening up before working the muscle.

5. If stretching a group of muscles affects another group (e.g., a thoracic stretch strains the shoulder joint), do not continue without further guidance.

6. After the muscle has been worked, stretch all muscle groups. Doing so is important in order to:

   a) Reduce bulking of the muscle;

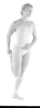

b) Reduce the risk of injury to joints, muscles, and tendons;

c) Reduce postexercise soreness in the muscle;

d) Maintain and increase joint mobility;

e) Increase flexibility;

f) Help you to cool down.

When starting any exercise routine, it is necessary to limber up before launching into the meat of the program. This can generally take the form of a five-minute bike ride, a jog around the block, or effective stretching that gradually lengthens and mobilizes the muscle groups for longer than ninety seconds at a time.

Gentle stretching can also form a part of this warm-up. This is especially true for those incapable of engaging in other methods of warming up, those who find other methods uncomfortable, or those with injuries. For those with an injury, stretching and strengthening the uninjured muscle groups by isolating them is an ideal means of staying in shape. As long as there are no effects on the injured muscles, tendons, joints, or ligaments, or on the area immediately surrounding the injury, exercising the uninjured muscles can keep the body toned and functioning and is much better than not exercising at all.

For the average person, substituting an extended stretching session for a warm-up routine is not detrimental. In fact, in some cases it is more beneficial and safer than other warm-up routines.

If the weather is cold, or if your muscles feel excessively tight, then you should spend extra time stretching. The time of day when you should stretch is entirely up to you. Some people feel much better stretching in the early morning (to wake themselves up), while others feel as if they are unable to move at all until the end of the working day, when the body has been mobilized and feels looser.

There is no evidence to suggest that practicing extended stretching techniques is detrimental to physical achievement when performing a controlled, nonstrenuous exercise program.

In order for the muscle to achieve its maximum range of movement, a continual stretch into the specific muscle area is required. Combined with the correct breathing technique (in through the nose for a count of five, followed with a sigh out through the mouth for a count of five, without depressing the chest), stretching helps to increase blood flow to the muscles. This greatly helps to improve the elasticity of the muscle as well as to eliminate lactic acid from the muscle group.

The Start Stretches (Exercises 3 through 6a) described at the beginning of this book's program are intended to stretch isolated muscle groups. The ideal order for stretching is to start with the back (lower and upper) and shoulders, continue with the hamstrings, and then move on to the thighs. Because some muscle groups are interdependent, stretching some muscles may reduce the need to stretch others. For example, stretching tight calves may reduce the need to stretch the hamstrings. Therefore, after stretching the back and shoulders, it would be prudent to stretch the calves before continuing with a hamstring stretch.

### HAIYONG R.

*While attempting a normal hamstring stretch, with the working leg resting on a bench and keeping the back in an upright position while holding onto the bench, Haiyong R. felt a cramping of the muscles in the middle back, just below the shoulder blades. This happened when he attempted to increase the forward lean and thereby to increase the stretch for the hamstring, which caused the latissimus dorsi and lower trapezium to grip. Haiyong R. was also found to be tightening the muscles between the shoulder blades (the rhomboids). These problems were easily corrected by depressing the shoulders and slightly rounding the upper back. The pain disappeared, and the effectiveness of the hamstring stretch was maintained.*

## POINTERS FOR SAFE EXERCISING

1. If at any time a stretch or exercise feels uncomfortable or painful, reduce its intensity by reducing the range of movement or easing the pressure on the joint.

2. If you feel sharp pain either in the part of the body being worked or in another part of the body, stop the exercise. Seek the advice of a qualified instructor on the movements you are doing.

3. If a movement feels too easy, first follow the principles and formula to enhance the quality of the movement, then increase the intensity of the exercise by progressing to the next version of the movement.

4. If you ever feel your neck straining during a supine exercise, support it with cushions or pillows. The exercise may then be completed without any strain on the breathing or on muscles that are not the working ones.

5. Whenever performing an exercise that requires you to be on your back, engage the B-Line Core and maintain the Stable Spine position unless otherwise stated in the instructions. If, as the exercise progresses, you feel that your back is arching, it may mean one of several things:

   a) Your legs may be too far away from the center. Draw the knees closer to the chest or bring the legs more vertically into the air.

   b) If the position requires the head and shoulders to be contracted forward (shoulder blades just off the floor, ribs to the hips and lined up in the same plane), you may be slowly releasing the contraction as the exercise progresses. Attempt to maintain the contraction at all times.

   c) The abdominal muscles may be gradually weakening, and the back muscles may be beginning to take over. If the back comes off the floor even one millimeter (if you can slide a ruler between your back and the floor), then the back may be doing more work than the abdominals. Stop the exercise. There is no point in continuing the exercise if the powerhouse muscles of the anatomy, the abdominals, are no longer supporting the movement.

6. Challenge yourself! Progress can be achieved only by increasing the intensity or range of movement of the exercise by a small percentage each time. Follow the program as closely as you can, and you will gain more confidence and body awareness. You will feel like a different person!

## THE STRUCTURE OF THE EXERCISE PROGRAM

The exercise program, which starts in the next chapter, is organized around the following general principles:

### 1. Prerequisite Exercises

In order to perform certain intermediate or advanced exercises comfortably and safely, it is necessary to first do some basic muscle strengthening or stretching. These prerequisite exercises are described at the beginning of the exercise section (in Chapter 5, "The Warm-Up").

### 2. Purpose of the Exercise/Muscles Worked

Each exercise includes a section describing the muscles that are to be worked and the purpose of the exercise. In several instances there is also an explanation of how the exercise relates to a "nonexercise" movement. This allows you to understand the practical use for what is being achieved in the routine and how the muscles being worked need to function outside of an exercise situation.

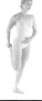

### 3. Description of the Exercise and Correct Breathing

The description of the exercise includes the following:

- Starting position—including engaging the B-Line or B-Line Core

- Back position—either Stable Spine or decompressing the spine (sometimes described in terms of the sacrum coin or lumbar coin)

- Breathing—starting the breath in or out slightly before the movement

- The steps or movements involved in the exercise itself

### 4. Key Points

There are major mental or physical points to consider when doing any movement. Slight variations in a movement, even it they are minor, can produce a considerable difference in the effectiveness of the exercise. Remember, even a centimeter's deviation in the placement of your body can mean up to 50 percent difference in the effectiveness of the exercise.

### 5. Repetitions

For each exercise, I suggest the ideal number of sets and repetitions. Remember that at the end of each repetition it is important to go on to the following repetition without resting, because if you rest, the muscle will relax and then will need to be reconnected or reengaged for the next repetition and may start out of alignment. One movement should flow into the next. At all times you should maintain muscle tone and muscle identification through isolation, as well as continuing to breathe deeply, using the ocean breath. By following these guidelines you can improve your mental and physical stamina and endurance, which will increase your confidence in what your body can achieve.

Complete only the number of repetitions with which you are comfortable. If you can manage only six repetitions before you start to feel that the ex-

ercise is no longer working properly or effectively, then stop after six. Add one repetition each week until you have reached the required number. (I have used the example of six repetitions because six is more than 50 percent of the generally required number of reps. By completing more than 50 percent, you will be closer to finishing and will have passed the psychological halfway barrier.)

The exercises are grouped into the following routines, with a chapter devoted to each. Careful thought has been given to people's differing abilities. If any of the exercises are too difficult, please follow the instructions outlined in the section "Pointers for Safe Exercising," above.

1. *The Warm-Up.* For loosening the tight major muscles of the legs, lower back, and shoulders.

2. *The Routine for Lower-Back Pain and Weak Abdominals.* For those who have minor lower-back pain that does not involve referred pain (pain going down the legs, etc.), and for those with weak abdominals.

3. *The Basic Routine.* For those starting an exercise program.

4. *The Intermediate Routine.* For those who have no back pain and are of a reasonable-to-average fitness level.

5. *The Advanced Routine.* For those who can complete the Intermediate Routine with ease, exercise regularly, and require a challenge.

6. *More Challenging Exercises.* For those who need a greater challenge than the advanced program.

7. *Theraband Routines.* For gaining strength with resistance.

Each routine is slightly more challenging than the one preceding it. If you feel that any exercise from a particular section is too difficult, substitute a similar exercise from a previous section. You may tailor your program to your own needs and abilities until you are able to follow the routines as suggested.

Alternatively, the book's final chapter, in the section titled "Increasing the Challenge: A Plan for Progressing Through the Exercises," offers another schedule for advancing through the exercises. The plan presented there is divided into several stages. Each week, add one more exercise from a stage until you are able to comfortably complete all the exercises in that stage. Then move on to the next stage.

Remember to seek medical approval or advice from a health-care professional or a qualified Pilates practitioner before embarking on any exercise program, especially if you have never attempted these exercises before.

I apologize in advance for the length of the explanations in some of the exercises. If at first you cannot understand the instructions well enough to make full use of them, do not worry. Start by following only two or three of the instructions for each exercise. As you become familiar and comfortable with these, then add another instruction. I feel it is better to give you as much information as possible, so that it will be available when you are ready to make full use of it. This not only provides you with the most comprehensive set of instructions ever written for Pilates exercises but should also answer all your questions in relation to the exercises.

You should wear snug but comfortable clothing. If possible, place a mirror where you can see yourself in order to correct any postural deviations that you would otherwise fail to notice. It would be ideal to have a friend read the instructions to you once you have a mental picture of what the exercise looks like from the photos or diagrams. For all the floor routines, use a thick but firm mat.

When embarking on the program, commit yourself to practicing it at least three times a week for six to eight weeks. The first two weeks will be the toughest. Any good, effective exercise program takes time to establish itself within your muscle memory. It took years to create the body you now have—it is not going to change overnight. Stick to it, and you will gradually start to see changes. You will be glad you persevered. Good luck!

# 5

# The Warm-Up

Not only is
health a normal
condition, but it
is a duty not only
to attain but to
maintain it.

— J. Pilates

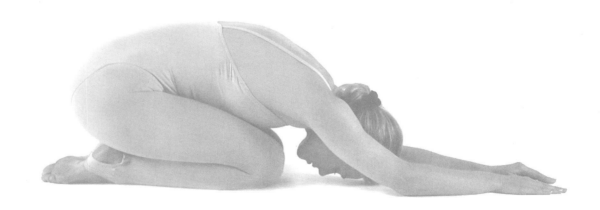

# Resting Position (Baby Pose)

**PREREQUISITE:** This position can be used at any time during the program.

**PURPOSE:** To relax and allow the spine to stretch and to mobilize the hips.

### EXERCISE DESCRIPTION:

*Starting Position:* Kneel back on your haunches, with your toes extended.

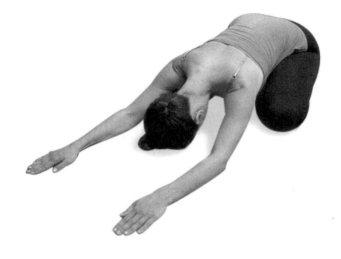

a) Keeping your buttocks on the heels as much as possible, slowly ocean breathe out to curl the spine forward while sliding your fingers out on the floor ahead of you.

b) Stretch all the way forward through your fingertips, while pressing your shoulder blades toward your hips. Rest your forehead and elbows on the floor. Breathe into the upper back and shoulder blades without moving.

c) Relax in this position.

**KEY POINTS:** On every breath out,

1. Press your buttocks onto your heels.

2. Lengthen your chest to your knees.

3. If you feel any discomfort in the knees, place a cushion behind the knees.

**REPETITIONS:** One set of ten breaths in and ten breaths out.

**BREATHING:** Breathe in and out deeply and slowly for ten breaths.

*Notes*

..............................................................

..............................................................

..............................................................

..............................................................

..............................................................

..............................................................

..............................................................

..............................................................

..............................................................

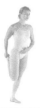

# Standing Roll Down

**PREREQUISITE:** This is a basic prerequisite for all exercises.

**PURPOSE:** To loosen up the spine, hamstrings, and lower back.

### EXERCISE DESCRIPTION:

*Starting position:* Stand as tall as you can with your feet shoulder distance apart and parallel. Imagine that your spine is stuck to a wall that takes the shape of your spine. Engage the B-Line Core, shoulders relaxed.

a) Bend your knees slightly, and ocean breathe out deeply to slowly and sequentially peel your vertebrae off the wall one at a time: start by lowering your chin forward to your rib cage, then ribs to hips, while pressing your lower back into the imaginary wall.

b) If you need to when you're halfway down, take a deep breath in, and then with a deep breath out, relax the body as far as it will comfortably go, keeping the knees slightly bent. If you cannot touch your toes, do not force yourself to do so. At the bottom of the movement, take a deep breath into the chest, maintaining the B-Line Core.

c) Ocean breathe out to return to the standing position, using your B-Line Core to imprint your spine onto the imaginary wall; or imagine stacking your vertebrae one on top of the other. The movement should be felt in the anterior (front) portion of the torso (the abdominals).

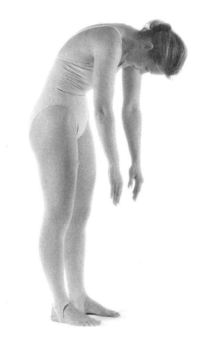

### KEY POINTS

1. Keep the body weight over the feet, which should be in the tripod position.

2. Lengthen the ribs away from the hips on the upward roll.

3. Squeeze the Core to come up; relax the shoulders.

4. If you feel the slightest strain in your back on the upward roll, bend the knees until only the abdominals are doing the work.

5. Only go down as far as you comfortably can.

**REPETITIONS:** One set of ten.

**BREATHING:** Ocean breathe out on the way down, breathe in at the point of flexion (relaxation), and ocean breathe out on the way up.

**INCREASE THE CHALLENGE:** Straighten the legs a bit more each time you do the movement.

# Stamina Stretch

**PREREQUISITE:** None.

**PURPOSE:** To increase lung capacity. To stretch the muscles down the side of the body, from the armpit to the hip.

### EXERCISE DESCRIPTION:

*Starting position:* Stand with your right side about eighteen inches away from a wall. Place the right hand against the wall at mid-thigh level, with the inside of the elbow facing the wall and the thumb pointing back. If the outside of the elbow faces the wall you will hunch the shoulder. Take the left hand over the head and place it against the wall at approximately head level, with the fingers facing backwards or down to the floor, depending on the flexibility in your shoulder joint.

a) Engage the B-Line Core. Ocean breathe out and stretch the outside hip away from the wall as far as possible. Straighten the top arm without sliding it up the wall.

b) Turn the navel slightly (about 20 percent) in toward the wall.

c) Stretch out further.

d) Strongly tuck the pelvis. You should feel an increase in the stretch between the outside rib and hip. Keep looking straight ahead, lengthening the crown of the head toward the wall.

e) Imagine someone's hand on your outside shoulder blade, and breathe into the shoulder blade as deeply as possible. Continue to breathe like this.

f) Turn the armpit or top elbow to the ceiling, keeping the hips in the slightly forward position.

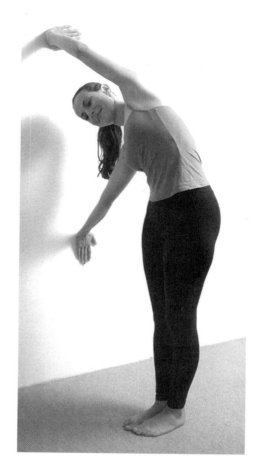

Repeat the breathing ten times. Then engage the B-Line Core to return to the upright position.

Before you change sides and repeat the movement, take a breath in and see how much extra lung capacity you have achieved in the left lung.

### KEY POINTS:

1. Relax the inside shoulder. Allow the head to relax, and look straight ahead.

2. Use the B-Line Core rather than the back muscles when returning to the upright position.

**REPETITIONS:** One set of ten breaths in and out per side.

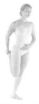

# The Start Stretches

**PREREQUISITE:** This is a basic prerequisite exercise for the whole program.

**PURPOSE:** To stretch the lower and middle back, and to open the groin area.

### EXERCISE DESCRIPTION:

*Starting Position:* Sit upright on the sitz bones as if against a wall, with feet drawn toward the groin, knees dropped open, and soles of the feet together. Ensure that the lowest six inches of the back are perfectly erect at all times. If they are not, place the feet farther away from the groin, or sit up against a wall and allow the spine to touch it without leaning against it at any time. The body should not be slumped into the hips. Sit as tall on the sitz bones as possible.

a) Reach the arms to the ceiling, stretching the spine; bend the elbows and place the fingers down the back between the shoulder blades. Imagine that you have suction cups on your finger tips, so as you curl forward the hands do not slide up toward the neck. This will increase the intensity of the stretch. Keep the shoulders relaxed when lifting the ribs from the hips.

b) Ocean breathe out to curl the head forward toward the chest (keeping a small space between your chin and your chest) and down toward the rib cage, letting the upper spine follow. You are attempting to roll your nose toward your B-Line, keeping the lowest six inches of the spine as upright as possible. This position will compress the chest, so breathe into the armpits (see "Breathing," in Chapter 2). Relax the knees open to the floor.

c) Hold the position for the breath in, without moving, then curl further forward toward the B-Line on the next breath out. Curl as far into the B-Line as possible on the first movement. After this the movements are very small, if at all.

This movement is very slight and can be felt quite strongly in the muscles on either side of the spine, in the lower back, or across the shoulder blades.

### KEY POINTS:

1. Keep the lumbar (lower) spine upright.

2. Lift out of the hips without hunching the shoulders.

3. Maintain the B-Line Core; keep elbows close to and behind the ears.

4. Relax the shoulders and neck; imagine that you're curving over a ball.

5. Sit tall on the sitz bones at all times; do not slump into the hips.

6. Keep the knees relaxed open.

7. If you feel as if you are rolling back onto the hips, place the feet farther away from the body until you are sitting tall comfortably.

8. To avoid any strain on the neck, do not cross the hands behind the head when curling forward.

9. Keep the chin softly off the chest.

**REPETITIONS:** One set of ten breaths in and ten out.

**BREATHING:** Breathe in while allowing the chest to expand through all areas, especially the armpits and upper back.

**VARIATIONS:** Sit tall on your sitz bones, and maintain the B-Line Core. Repeat the exercise as above, moving the feet to the different positions described below (Exercises 4 through 6a) for the ten-breath repetition.

# The Start Stretches *(cont'd.)*

**DURATION:** Ten slow breaths in and out, contracting farther forward on each breath out.

## Exercise 4

Extend your legs straight in front of you, keeping them together, with your feet pointed. Make sure your knees are pointing up to the ceiling so the thighs are not turned out. Press the ankle bones together. If the feeling is too strong behind the knees, bend the knees only slightly.

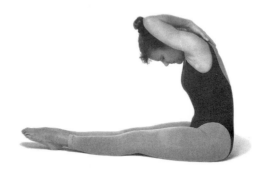

## Exercise 5

Extend your legs straight in front of you, keeping them together, with your feet flexed and pressing through the heels. Knees are pointing toward the ceiling, as in Exercise 4. This stretch should be felt comfortably in the spine and mildly to strongly in the hamstrings.

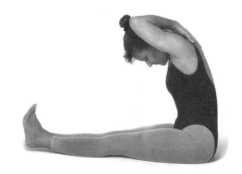

## Exercise 6

Extend the left leg straight in front of the left hip, knee pointed toward ceiling, foot flexed. Bend the right leg at the knee and place the sole of the right foot against the inside of the left knee. The hips should be square and the leg in line with the hip. Do not adjust the hips to establish the position—only adjust the legs.

## Exercise 6a

Reverse the legs and repeat Exercise 6.

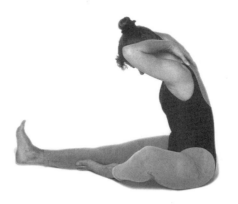

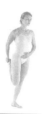

# Spiral Stretch

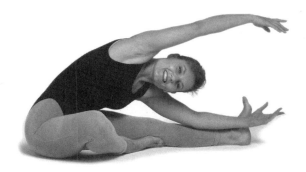

**PREREQUISITE:** To be able to perform upper-back stretches correctly, with no problems or strain in the back whatsoever. To be able to line up the sternum (breastbone) with the bent knee. Note: Do not perform this stretch if you have any back problems or back pain.

**PURPOSE:** To stretch the sides between the armpit and the hips, the lower-back muscles, and the shoulder joints.

### EXERCISE DESCRIPTION:

*Starting Position:* Sit as in Exercise 6 (left leg straight, right leg bent). Breathe in and reach both arms to the ceiling.

a) Engage the B-Line Core and rotate the torso to the right, rotating the center of the breastbone (sternum) until it is in line with or past the point of the bent knee.

b) Ocean breathe out to stretch the torso sideways along the extended leg. Hold onto the foot or the ankle of the straight leg with the left hand.

c) Breathe in without moving. Ocean breathe out to bend the left elbow and to lengthen the left armpit toward the left knee (without bending the knee). Stretch the right hand past the left foot and parallel to the floor. Breathe in without moving. Repeat ten times.

d) To finish, lengthen both arms past the extended foot, squeeze the B-Line Core, and breathe in to reach out of the hips toward the ceiling (remaining rotated); then rotate back to the front position. Relax the hands by the sides. Change sides.

### KEY POINTS:

1. Keep the hips square, maintaining the B-Line Core.

2. Keep both sitz bones on the floor, or press the opposite hip to the floor.

3. Lengthen through the spine, with the uppermost armpit to the ceiling, and avoid overarching in the lower back; maintain the top arm/elbow behind the top ear.

4. The more rotation and lengthening you can achieve, the better the stretch.

5. Keep the body directly over the extended leg and slightly in front of it for a better stretch.

**REPETITIONS:** Breathe in ten times and ocean breathe out ten times. Do one set on each side.

**BREATHING:** Breathe in to hold the position; ocean breathe out to stretch over the extended leg.

**INCREASE THE CHALLENGE:** If you are flexible enough to hold the foot of the extended leg with the top hand, do so. Place the other hand on the floor past the bent knee. When breathing out, bend the elbow of the top hand to the ceiling, holding onto the foot for leverage, and walk the fingers of the bottom hand along the floor past the bent knee. On every breath out, rotate and lengthen the torso further. We call this the Pretzel Stretch. Press the hip of the bent leg into the floor for a better stretch. Maintain the B-Line Core at all times.

# Calf Stretch

**PREREQUISITE:** None.

**PURPOSE:** To stretch and strengthen the calf muscles (gastrocnemius and soleus).

### EXERCISE DESCRIPTION:

*Starting Position:* Stand with the balls of the feet on the edge of a step. Place a tennis ball between the ankles to prevent the feet from rolling outward on the rise. Place a thick pad between the knees to prevent them from rolling in and to help to connect (engage) the inner thigh muscles.

   a) Engage the B-Line Core with a slight tuck of the pelvis. Breathe in to rise up onto the balls of the feet as high as possible. Keep the tennis ball between the ankles. Think of working the muscles in the feet rather than working from the calves.

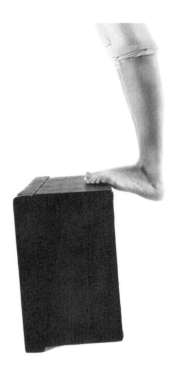

   b) Ocean breathe out to lower the heels below the level of the step, pressing the heels down as far as possible. As the heels lower below the horizontal level, squeeze the pad and lightly turn out the upper thighs. The knees and upper thighs have a tendency to roll in at this point.

### KEY POINTS:

1. Do not drop the ball or the pad.

2. If the knees are too far apart, use a thicker pad.

3. The point of the rise should be mainly (70 percent) on the ball of the big toe (tripod position 1, see page 35).

4. Do not allow the lower back to arch at any time. If necessary, tuck your pelvis slightly to prevent this.

5. Do not drop into the heels; lower and press down gradually.

**REPETITIONS:** Fifteen to twenty repetitions.

*Notes*

........................................................

........................................................

........................................................

........................................................

........................................................

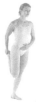

# Alternating Calf Stretches

**PREREQUISITE:** Exercise 8-1.

**PURPOSE:** To stretch the calves more than in the previous exercise, especially if one calf is tighter than the other.

### EXERCISE DESCRIPTION:

*Starting Position:* Stand on the edge of a step on the balls of the feet. Engage the B-Line Core, and breathe in to rise up onto the balls of the feet (tripod position 1, see page 35) as high as possible.

a) Ocean breathe out to lower the right heel below the level of the step, while the left leg stays high on the ball of the foot, bending the left knee. Slightly turn out the right thigh to prevent the knee from rolling in.

b) Breathe in to rise up on the right foot, only to the height of the left foot. Change feet and repeat with the left foot.

**KEY POINTS:** As in Exercise 8-1. In addition,

1. Use the muscles of only one foot at a time.

2. Do not let the hips swing out to the sides by sinking into them.

**REPETITIONS:** Twenty repetitions, alternating legs.

**VARIATION FOR THE SOLEUS:** As the heel lowers below the horizontal position, bend the knee to stretch the soleus (the deeper layer of the calf muscles).

*Notes*

.................................................

.................................................

.................................................

.................................................

.................................................

.................................................

.................................................

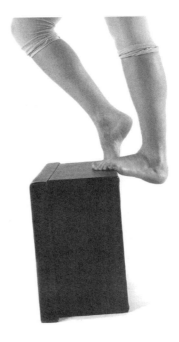

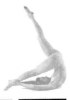

# Hamstring Stretch: Basic

**PREREQUISITE:** This is a basic prerequisite exercise.

**PURPOSE:** To safely stretch the hamstring muscles for those with extremely tight hamstrings or with back pain.

### EXERCISE DESCRIPTION:

*Starting Position:* Lie on your back with the knees bent at a right angle. Feet are flat on the floor. Decompress the spine.

a) Bend one knee to the chest and place a long towel or strap around the heel.

b) Slowly extend the heel to the ceiling while holding on to the towel. Keep extending the foot until you feel a strong stretch in the hamstring (not behind the knee). If the leg fully extends and there is no effect on the spine, move on to Exercise 9-2.

c) Breathe in to hold the position.

d) Ocean breathe out to press the heel toward the wall above the crown of the head for more of a stretch, at the same time pressing that hip into the floor.

### KEY POINTS:

1. Maintain the B-Line Core.

2. Keep the hips firmly pressed to the floor, as though you're pressing the sacrum coin down.

3. Place a cushion under the head if the neck arches; keep the eyes on the knee of the stretching leg.

4. Press the elbows slightly away from the sides of the body and toward the foot that's on the floor.

5. Keep the shoulder blades pressed into the pocket.

**REPETITIONS:** Ten breaths in and ten breaths out. Do two sets on each leg, alternating legs. It is important to alternate the legs rather than doing all twenty repetitions without stopping. This gives the muscle some time to relax before subjecting it to more stretching. By doing this you avoid pushing the muscle to its limits without a break. Therefore, you get more benefit from the exercise, because you are able to do a better conscious stretch during the second set.

**BREATHING:** Ocean breathe out to press through the heel. Breathe in to hold the position.

**INCREASE THE CHALLENGE:** As the exercise becomes easier, slowly straighten the bent leg. Continue to draw the leg being stretched toward the same shoulder, without bending the knee. As the stretched leg is able to maintain a straight position, gradually extend the leg on the mat to an almost straight position, keeping the lumbar coin pressed down into the floor and flexing the foot.

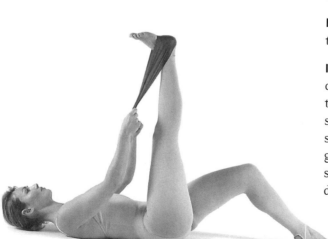

# Hamstring Stretch 2

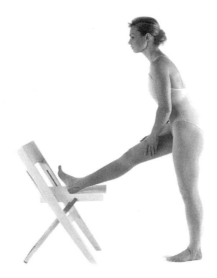

**PREREQUISITE:** Stretched calves (Exercises 8-1 and 8-2).

**PURPOSE:** To perform a more specific stretch on the hamstring group.

### EXERCISE DESCRIPTION:

*Starting Position:* Standing upright, place the right foot on a chair or table, with the upper leg raised to hip level. If you are more flexible, you can raise the leg higher. Your left foot should be facing forward.

a) Keep the hips square and parallel, the right foot flexed, and the right kneecap pointed to the ceiling. Engage the B-Line Core.

b) Keep the right knee as straight as possible, without locking (hyperextending) it. Look straight ahead. Maintain the B-Line Core and ocean breathe out to lean your ribs forward to a point at about eye-level. Imagine that on every breath out, you are growing taller as you lean forward out of the hips. Do not bend the head or chest to the knee. Keep the head upright at all times, stretching through the crown of the head to the ceiling.

c) Hold the position for the breath in; ocean breathe out to lift and lean forward farther (only a slight movement is required).

### KEY POINTS:

1. If you feel more pressure behind the knee than in the hamstring, bend the knee.

2. Imagine that someone is lifting you out of your lower back: lift up and away from the tailbone, almost as if you were attempting to arch the very lowest part of the back.

3. Keep the pelvis square and level to the floor.

4. Keep the supporting leg firmly planted into the floor directly below the hip at all times. Press through the heel as much as possible to achieve more stretch.

5. Constantly maintain the B-Line Core.

6. If you feel tightness between the shoulder blades, round the shoulders slightly.

7. If you feel a mild tightness in the lower back, bend slightly forward from the lower back.

8. Keep the hips square and level, keep the supporting leg directly under the hip, and be sure to avoid hyperextending the knee.

9. On the stretch scale, this should register no greater than 8.5 in the hamstring and only slightly behind the knee.

**REPETITIONS:** Breathe in and out ten times.

**BREATHING:** Breathe in to lengthen the spine to the ceiling, and ocean breathe out to lean the ribs to the wall at eye level. Remain in this posture for ten breaths. On each out breath, extend farther up and forward to feel the stretch.

# Hamstring Stretch 3

a) Sit on one leg on a flat bench. In this position it is easier to keep the hips level. The leg on the ground is bent and the toes are facing forward. This is easier than the version above.

b) Use the hands to lean the body farther forward by holding on to the leg or the bench and bending at the elbows.

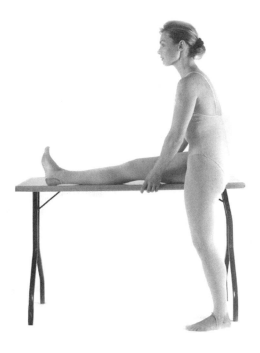

*Notes*

.................................................

.................................................

.................................................

.................................................

.................................................

.................................................

.................................................

.................................................

.................................................

.................................................

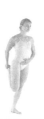

# Thigh Stretch 1: Prone

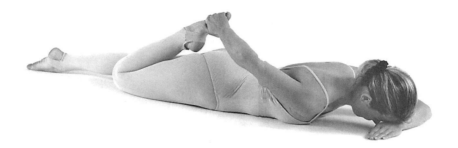

**PREREQUISITE:** This is a basic prerequisite exercise for those who cannot do Thigh Stretches 2 or 3.

**PURPOSE:** To stretch the thigh-muscle group, especially for those with knee problems.

### EXERCISE DESCRIPTION:

*Starting Position:* Lie face-down on a mat with a small, folded towel placed under the stomach between the ribs and the hips, to assist in maintaining the B-Line. Bend the right leg, drawing the foot to the buttock. Reach back with the right hand and grasp the foot. The body should remain in a straight line, without the shoulders twisting or the knee shifting away from a straight line with the hip. You should feel a mild to strong stretch along the front of the right thigh.

Ocean breathe out to bend the right elbow in order to bring the heel closer to the buttock, maintaining the B-Line Core and pressing the right hipbone to the floor. Hold the position for the breath in. Repeat ten times, drawing the heel closer to the buttock each time.

### KEY POINTS:

1. The towel is meant to help prevent the back from arching and reduce any pressure in the lower back.

2. If you are able to place the hipbone flat on the floor, then progress to Thigh Stretch 2, as long as you have no knee problems.

3. If you cannot bend the knee to the buttock comfortably, place a towel around the foot, hold on to the towel, and draw the foot toward the buttock.

**REPETITIONS:** One set of ten breaths, alternating.

**BREATHING:** Ten breaths in and ten breaths out in each set.

### Notes

..........................................................................

..........................................................................

..........................................................................

..........................................................................

..........................................................................

# Thigh Stretch 2: Standing

**PREREQUISITE:** This is a basic prerequisite exercise.

**PURPOSE:** To stretch the thighs and open the lower back.

### EXERCISE DESCRIPTION:

*Starting Position:* To stretch the left thigh, stand with the right leg on the floor and the left leg bent on a chair, or hold on to the left foot with the left hand. This requires some balance. Your balance will improve over time as you complete more stretches.

a) Ocean breathe out to tuck the pelvis under. This can be greatly assisted by pressing the left buttock toward the floor and drawing the pubic bone toward the rib cage with the assistance of the right hand.

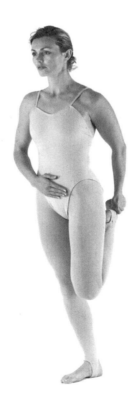

b) Breathe into the position and hold. Ocean breathe out to tuck the pelvis under even more.

### KEY POINTS:

1. Remain leaning slightly forward all the time. This opens the lower back, and the continual tuck opens it even further.

2. Ensure that the hips are level and square before you start the exercise.

3. Ensure that the front of the thighs are level with each other. If the thigh being stretched is farther forward than the (other) supporting leg, press the knee down toward the floor as much as possible while bringing it in line with the supporting leg, without arching the back. This should induce a stronger stretch with a small movement of the thigh downward.

4. Press the elbows toward the floor.

5. The thigh stretch is the only one on which you may reach level 9 (out of 10) on the stretch scale.

**REPETITIONS:** One set of ten breaths in and ten breaths out, alternating legs.

**BREATHING:** Breathe in without moving; ocean breathe out to tuck the pelvis.

*Notes*

. . . . . . . . . . . . . . . . . . . . . . . . . . . . . . . . . . . . . . . . . . . . . . . .

. . . . . . . . . . . . . . . . . . . . . . . . . . . . . . . . . . . . . . . . . . . . . . . .

. . . . . . . . . . . . . . . . . . . . . . . . . . . . . . . . . . . . . . . . . . . . . . . .

# Thigh Stretch 3: Kneeling

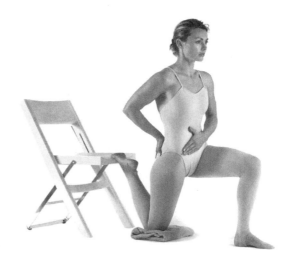

**PREREQUISITE:** Achieving Thigh Stretch 2 without feeling much strain.

**PURPOSE:** To stretch the thigh muscles and iliopsoas, connect the B-Line Core, and open the lower back. (The iliopsoas is the muscle that attaches from the lower spine to the top of the thigh bone. If the abdominals are weak, this muscle tends to arch the lower back.)

### EXERCISE DESCRIPTION:

*Starting Position:* To stretch the right thigh, place a thick towel or a piece of dense foam under the right knee. Then place the hands on the floor, bend the right knee, and put the right foot against a wall or on a chair. If this is uncomfortable on the front of the foot, place a soft pad under the foot. Bend the left knee, place both hands on the left knee, and come into an upright position.

a) The exercise now follows the same steps as Thigh Stretch 2.

b) Place the right hand on the right buttock and the left hand just above the pubic bone. Press the buttock toward the floor and draw the pubic bone toward the rib cage.

### KEY POINTS:

1. Make sure that the hips are not thrust forward, as this can arch the spine and put pressure on the lower back.

2. Maintain the B-Line Core. This will assist in a stronger stretch.

3. Keep the foot of the supporting leg at a right angle to the knee so no undue pressure is placed on the toes. Use the tripod position (see page 35) for the supporting foot.

4. You can increase the stretch by pressing with the hands to enhance the tuck, as the muscles may be too tight to achieve this on their own.

5. To achieve an even greater stretch, imagine that the hipbone of the leg being stretched is drawing strongly up toward the rib cage on that side.

6. The closer the knee is to the wall, the better the stretch.

7. If you feel any pain in the knee joint, stop and try Exercise 11.

8. Keep the hand on the buttock only, not on the lower back.

**REPETITIONS:** Two sets of ten breaths and ten breaths out, alternating legs.

**BREATHING:** Hold the position on the breath in; ocean breathe out to tuck the pelvis.

# Thigh Stretch 3: Kneeling *(cont'd.)*

**INCREASE THE CHALLENGE:**

If you feel only a minimal stretch, try the following:

1. Place the supporting leg farther forward, and lean the entire body forward away from the wall and heel. Without arching the back, tuck the pelvis. You will feel the stretch higher up the thigh, toward the hipbone.

2. If this is too easy, stay in the forward-leaning position, reach back, and grasp the foot, pulling gently away from the wall toward the buttock. Try to maintain the tuck without arching the back. This should induce an extremely strong stretch toward the top of the thigh. Keep the shoulders square.

# 6

## The Routine for Lower-Back Pain and Weak Abdominals

Be in control

of your body—

*not* at its mercy.

— UNKNOWN

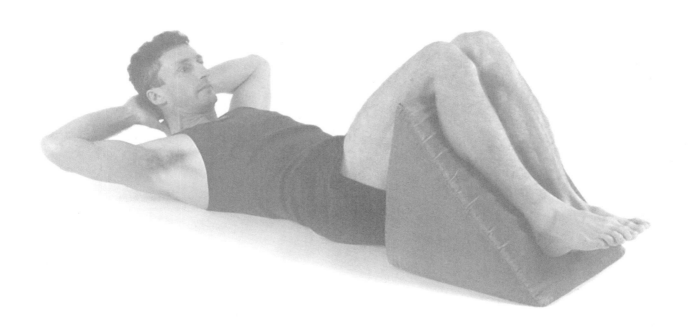

# One-Leg Lifts: Supine

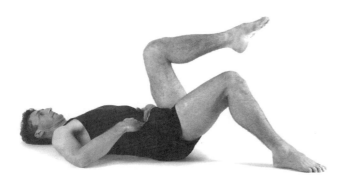

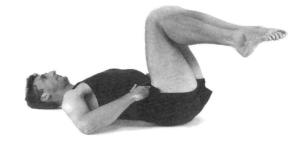

**PREREQUISITES:** Warm-up stretches.

**PURPOSE:** To achieve basic strength for the lower abdominals.

### EXERCISE DESCRIPTION:

*Starting Position:* Lie on your back (supine) with the feet flat on the floor and the knees bent at forty-five degrees. Decompress the spine. Engage the B-Line Core and maintain the Stable Spine. Place your fingers on the insides of the hipbones. Press firmly.

a) Breathe out to draw the right knee toward your chest, keeping the right buttock on the ground. Do not place any pressure on the floor with the left foot. As the right foot is lifted off the floor, you may feel the abdominals push up against the fingers. Draw the abdominals in as hard as you can away from the fingers by squeezing the B-Line Core.

b) Breathe in to hold the leg toward you, then ocean breathe out to slowly lower the leg to the floor, still squeezing the Core.

**KEY POINTS:**

1. Ocean breathe out to lower the leg.

2. At the same time, flatten the rib cage to the floor.

3. If the lower back arches when the leg lifts, place the foot of the stationary leg on a chair.

**REPETITIONS:** Ten on each leg, alternating after each repetition.

**INCREASE THE CHALLENGE:** Attempt the same abdominal connection while either extending one leg straight on the ground or drawing both knees to the chest at the same time, without allowing the back to arch.

*Notes*

. . . . . . . . . . . . . . . . . . . . . . . . . . . . . . . . . . . . . . . . . . .

. . . . . . . . . . . . . . . . . . . . . . . . . . . . . . . . . . . . . . . . . . .

. . . . . . . . . . . . . . . . . . . . . . . . . . . . . . . . . . . . . . . . . . .

. . . . . . . . . . . . . . . . . . . . . . . . . . . . . . . . . . . . . . . . . . .

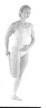

# Sliding Leg

**PREREQUISITES:** Warm-up stretches.

**PURPOSE:** To maintain the abdominal connection when the body is lengthening.

### EXERCISE DESCRIPTION:

*Starting Position:* Lie on your back with legs bent (feet flat on the floor) and fingers placed on the lower abdominals. Press firmly. Draw the abdominal muscles in, away from the fingers. Engage the B-Line Core.

a) Ocean breathe out to bend one leg up to your chest, slowly straightening the other leg by sliding the foot along the floor away from the torso, intensifying the squeeze on the Core.

b) Breathe in to slowly extend the raised leg away from the chest and back toward the floor, still squeezing the Core and drawing the abdominals away from your fingers.

### KEY POINTS:

1. Imagine that the abdominal muscles are connected to the thigh and that they are drawing in tighter as you draw the leg toward you. As the leg extends away from you, squeeze the Core and flatten the rib cage.

2. Do not tighten the buttocks.

3. On the breaths in and out, flatten the ribs toward the floor, breathing into the armpits.

4. Keep the neck lengthened and the shoulders relaxed. If the neck is arched, place a small cushion under the head.

**REPETITIONS:** Ten on each leg, alternating legs after each repetition.

### INCREASE THE CHALLENGE:

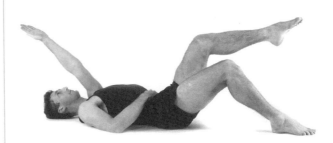

*More Challenging:* Start with the right arm on the floor above the head. Breathe in to draw the right leg toward you, while raising the right arm to the ceiling. Then, breathe out to lower both the arm and the leg to the floor while maintaining the B-Line Core and Stable Spine and flattening the rib cage to the floor.

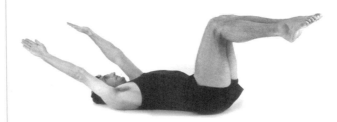

*Even More Challenging:* Repeat the preceding variation, but move both arms and both legs together, trying to control any arch in the back by maintaining the B-Line Core and flattening the rib cage on the breath out (extension of the body).

# Sliding Leg *(cont'd.)*

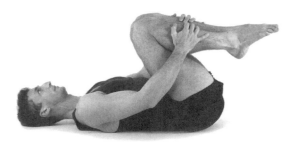

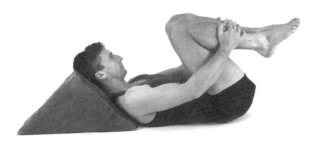

## Rest Position with Knees to Chest for Exercises Done while Lying on the Back

Lie on your back on a comfortable mat. Decompress the spine. Draw the knees to the chest and place the hands on the knees, drawing the heels into the tailbone and keeping the sacrum pressed onto the imaginary coin. Lengthen the neck and press the shoulder blades into the pocket. This is the standard position for the start of most exercises that progress to a contraction position (ribs to hips, head forward, shoulder blades off the ground, arms forward past the hips at mid-thigh level).

## Position for All Exercises with Cushion

Place your head on a large cushion or several pillows with the bottom of the shoulder blades at the junction of the floor and the cushion. There should be no gap between the back and the floor at any time during the exercise, especially if the arms are raised into the air or behind the head. The head, neck, and chin should be comfortable, with at least a golf-ball-size space between the chin and the chest at all times. If the knees are raised vertically, the eyes should be focused on the knees.

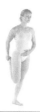

THE ROUTINE FOR LOWER-BACK PAIN AND WEAK ABDOMINALS

# Preparation with Cushions

**PREREQUISITES:** Warm-up stretches.

**PURPOSE:** To strengthen and gain control of the abdominals and to feel the entire abdominal section working.

### EXERCISE DESCRIPTION:

*Starting Position:* Lying on the cushion, decompress the spine. Draw the knees to the chest and hold on to them lightly with your hands.

a) Ocean breathe out to extend the hands forward past the hips at mid-thigh level while extending the legs vertically into the air.

b) Engage the B-Line and draw the ribs to the hips.

c) Breathe in to return to the starting position.

### KEY POINTS:

1. Keep the eyes focused on the knees.

2. Be sure to let out an ocean breath.

3. The B-Line should be connected firmly while scooping the abdominals for greater effect and support for the lower back.

4. Raise the legs only as high as you can while still keeping the lumbar coin pressed into the floor.

**REPETITIONS:** Do ten repetitions. When you first do the exercise, rest for half a second between each repetition to gain continual tone in the muscle. As you become more proficient at the exercise, do not rest at all.

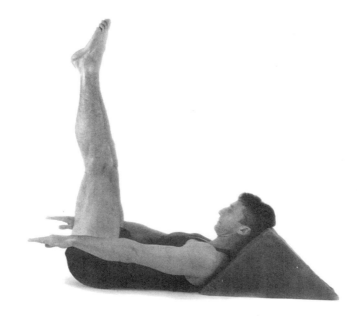

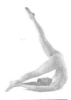

# 7

Remember, too, that "Rome was not built in a day," and that patience and persistence are vital qualities in the ultimate successful accomplishment of any worthwhile endeavor.

— J. PILATES

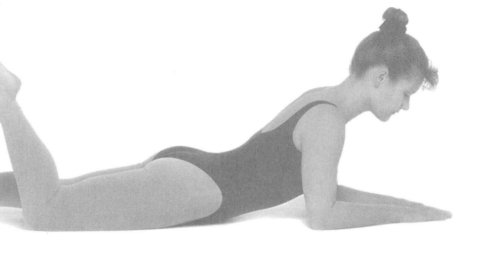

# Preparation for the Hundreds

**PREREQUISITES:** Warm-up stretches.

**PURPOSE:** Abdominal work to control and reduce overarching in the lower back.

### EXERCISE DESCRIPTION:

***Starting Position:*** Lie supine on the floor with the arms above the head and the legs together, toes pointed, squeezing the inner thighs together (Figure i).

a) Breathe in to raise the arms to the ceiling and bend the knees, sliding the toes on the ground (Figure ii).

b) Engage the B-Line, and ocean breathe out to contract forward, extending the arms past the hips at mid-thigh level and raising the legs vertically (Figure iii).

c) Breathe in to raise the arms vertically and bend the knees so the toes touch the floor, keeping your torso contracted forward.

d) Ocean breathe out to extend the arms, head, and legs on the floor to the starting position.

### KEY POINTS:

1. Stretch through the fingertips, palms facing down.

2. Slide the toes along the floor, keeping the heels off the floor and squeezing the inner thighs together strongly.

3. Keep the shoulders pressed into the pocket.

4. Keep the rhythm smooth during the movement.

5. If the neck starts to strain, put cushions under the head and take the arms back only as far as is comfortable.

**REPETITIONS:** Ten repetitions.

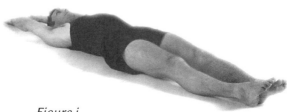

*Figure i*

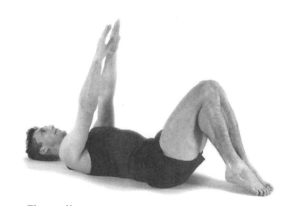

*Figure ii*

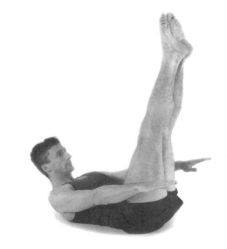

*Figure iii*

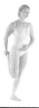

# The Hundreds: Basic

**PREREQUISITES:** The Start Stretches (Exercises 3 through 6a).

**PURPOSE:** To strengthen the abdominal muscles.

### EXERCISE DESCRIPTION:

*Starting Position:* Lying on your back, decompress the spine, with knees to your chest and hands relaxed on the knees.

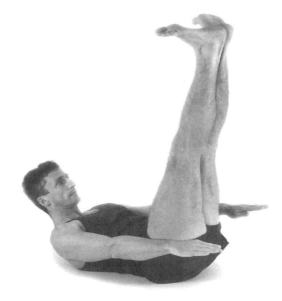

a) Engage B-Line and ocean breathe out to contract forward. Extend the hands forward past the hips at mid-thigh level, stretching through the fingertips, palms down.

b) Raise your legs vertically into the air, flexing your feet and rotating your legs outward from the inner thighs. Squeeze the backs of the knees together to engage the adductors (this will take the pressure off the front of the thighs). Pinch the buttocks slightly.

c) Keeping the eyes on the knees and maintaining the B-Line, breathe in for a five count and then ocean breathe out for a five count. Repeat ten breaths in and out without resting. (The ten counts in and out for ten repetitions equals one hundred—hence, the name The Hundreds.)

### KEY POINTS:

1. Keep the rib cage drawn as closely as possible to the hips at all times, shoulder blades off the mat and eyes on the knees.

2. If the shoulders drop back on the breath in, contract farther forward on the breath in.

3. Scoop the abdominals. If you do not feel the abdominals while doing this exercise, then attempt the intermediate Hundreds (Exercise 19-1).

4. If the back arches or strains, turn the legs in and bend the knees slightly, keeping the heels in a vertical line with the buttocks.

5. If you feel the neck strain, place a cushion under the head, and raise the head on each breath out only. Scoop the abdominals when releasing to the cushion. As the neck becomes stronger, raise the head up for two breaths, and so on.

6. To assist in maintaining the B-Line, place a small weight on the lower abdominals and draw the abdominals away from the weight, especially on the breath in. When the weight no longer moves, remove it.

**REPETITIONS:** Two sets of ten breaths in and ten breaths out. Take no more than a ten-second rest between each set.

# The Hundreds: Intermediate

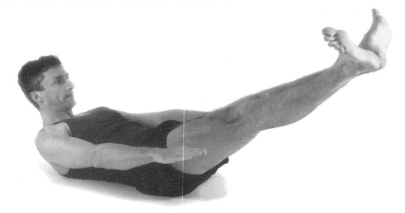

**PREREQUISITES:** Warm-up stretches and the ability to do two sets of basic Hundreds comfortably.

**PURPOSE:** To strengthen the abdominals by moving the body's center of gravity.

**EXERCISE DESCRIPTION:** Start in the same position as for the basic Hundreds. Lower the legs until you feel that the imaginary lumbar coin is just about to lift off the mat, making sure the abdominals do not rise even one millimeter (think of a greyhound's stomach—the dog, not the bus!). Engage the B-Line strongly. Breathe in ten times and out ten times.

### KEY POINTS:

1. The back must remain flat throughout the exercise, keeping the imaginary lumbar coin pressed into the mat.

2. Allow the shoulder blades to lift no higher than just off the floor, and keep them there at all times.

3. If the abdominals rise higher than the level of the hips and ribs, raise the legs higher and scoop the stomach.

4. Scoop the B-Line on the breath in.

**REPETITIONS:** Two sets of ten breaths.

**INCREASE THE CHALLENGE:** To engage the lower abdominals more specifically, even while maintaining the B-Line, keep the legs at a low angle while pressing the lumbar coin into the floor. Without moving the angle of the legs, try to lift your sacrum off the floor. It will not actually lift a noticeable distance, but you should feel the immediate, strong connection of the lower abdominals. Maintain this position for the whole set.

*Notes*

..........................................................

..........................................................

..........................................................

..........................................................

..........................................................

..........................................................

..........................................................

# Percussion Breathing

This exercise is more advanced when you are able to keep the abdominals scooped at all times. It follows the same routine as the preceding one, with the following addition: Keep the knees facing upward (rather than turned out), with the toes softly pointed. When the hands are extended beyond the hips and positioned about six inches off the floor, pump the hands up and down a few inches, moving from about mid-thigh level to the knees and back again. Each pump should take half a second. Do "percussion" breaths in for five pumps of the arms (in, in, in, in, in) and five percussion breaths out for five pumps (out, out, out, out, out). One pump is a single up and down movement of the arms. Do not stop the breathing or pumping at any time until you have completed one hundred pumps of the arms. Keeping the hands high allows ease of breathing and releases the pectorals. It also keeps the B-Line connected more strongly.

Alternative: Instead of a smooth five seconds of breathing in, the breathing should be done as five individual breaths in (or out) until full capacity (or deflation) is achieved. That is, expel (or take in) a little bit of air with the first pump of the hands, a little bit more with the second pump of the hands, and so on. This gives a percussion effect to the breathing, and it can increase the effect on the abdominals. The breathing is almost as if you are coughing each breath out. Squeeze a thin pad between the knees for even more abdominal effect.

KEY POINTS: If you find that this exercise is straining the neck rather than connecting strongly in the abdominals, revert to the basic Hundreds until the abdominals are stronger.

*Notes*

# Single Leg Stretch

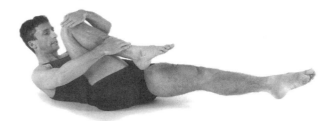

**PREREQUISITES:** The Start Stretches (Exercises 3 through 6a).

**PURPOSE:** To mobilize the hip and knee joints, control the abdominals, and increase coordination.

### EXERCISE DESCRIPTION:

*Starting Position:* Lie flat on your back, with both knees to the chest. Decompress the spine.

a) Ocean breathe out to contract forward, placing the right hand on the right ankle and the left hand on the right knee, elbows raised and extended forward.

b) Extend the left leg away from the body in line with the hip and as low to the floor as possible, pressing the imaginary lumbar coin into the mat. As the leg extends, turn it out and stretch through the point of the foot.

c) Engage the B-Line and scoop the stomach. Breathe in to change legs, keeping the outside hand on the corresponding ankle (left hand, left ankle), and draw the left knee to the left shoulder.

### KEY POINTS:

1. Keep the shoulders relaxed, chin slightly off the chest.

2. Engage the B-Line before changing legs.

3. Keep the ribs drawn as close to the hips as possible.

4. Use the hands as a guide only; do not use them to pull on the leg or to hunch the shoulder.

5. When extending the leg, feel as if the inner thighs were squeezing a cushion.

6. When extending the leg from the bent position, stretch through the toe along the line of the leg's final position, like the action of a piston (i.e., do not extend the leg into the air and then lower it to the ground as though you were pedaling a bicycle).

7. Keep the shoulders square at all times by pressing both elbows toward the hips.

8. Keep the eyes on the long knee.

9. If the neck starts to strain, place a cushion under the head and shoulders.

**REPETITIONS:** One set of ten repetitions, alternating legs.

**VARIATIONS:** Instead of holding on with the hands, place the wrists over the knee and ankle, with the fingers extended to the far walls. This action will ease the knee closer to the shoulder and reduce any excessive neck and shoulder work.

**INCREASE THE CHALLENGE:** After six repetitions, straighten and extend the arms past the hips at mid-thigh level, and continue to alternate the legs. Try to draw the knees back as close to the shoulders as before, on their own. Repeat for ten repetitions. Feel the B-Line connect strongly.

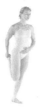

# Double Leg Stretch: Basic

*This exercise may appear confusing because of the amount of instruction. Please persevere; it will be worth it!*

**PREREQUISITES:** Preparation for the Hundreds (Exercise 17), The Hundreds: Basic (Exercise 18).

**PURPOSE:** To strengthen the abdominals while moving the body's center of gravity. To mobilize the shoulder joints. To coordinate breathing and arm and leg movement with abdominal control.

### EXERCISE DESCRIPTION:

*Starting Position:* Lie on your back on the floor, knees comfortably bent to the chest and slightly apart, feet flexed, heels squeezed together, and hands on the knees or shins (whichever avoids hunching the shoulders). Decompress the spine. Draw the heels to the buttocks. Place your head on a cushion if required (Figure i).

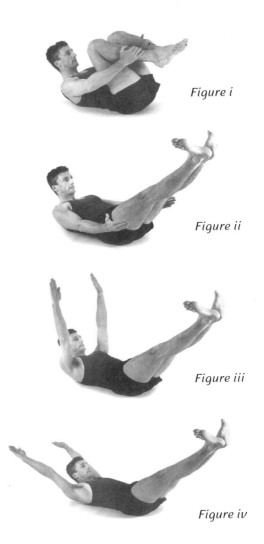

*Figure i*

*Figure ii*

*Figure iii*

*Figure iv*

a) Engage the B-Line and ocean breathe out to contract forward. Extend the arms forward past the hips at mid-thigh level, stretching through the fingertips. On the same breath out, extend the legs away from the torso, with the feet flexed and the legs turned out, keeping the legs as low to the floor as is comfortable. Keep the imaginary lumbar coin pressed into the floor, and scoop the stomach. Press through the heels, and squeeze the inner thighs together (Figure ii).

b) Breathe in to extend the arms to a vertical position, reaching through the fingers toward the ceiling; don't hunch the shoulders. Hold the position for one second and engage the B-Line even more firmly (Figure iii).

c) Maintaining the B-Line, ocean breathe out to lower the arms toward the ground be-

hind the head, grazing the ears with the upper arms. Then move the arms in a big circle around and back to their starting position with hands next to hips, palms down. Imagine that the arms are floating through this entire movement. Draw the ribs toward the hips even more tightly, keeping the legs and the upper torso in their slightly elevated positions. All of this step is done on a single breath out (Figure iv).

# Double Leg Stretch: Basic *(cont'd.)*

d) Breathe in to return to your starting position. Rest for only half a second before repeating the movement.

### KEY POINTS:

1. As the arms move from the vertical position to behind the head, ensure that the ribs stay drawn toward the hips. This movement should always be done on a breath out, depressing the rib cage.

2. Press through the heels as much as you can.

3. Rotate the legs outward as much as possible from the inner thighs. Stretch through the tips of the fingers at all times, making sure not to hunch the shoulders.

4. Do not allow the shoulder blades to lower to the floor on the arm circle; if this happens, contract farther forward.

5. If the neck feels any pressure, keep the head on a high cushion at all times.

6. If the back begins to arch after several movements, raise the legs to a higher position so that the imaginary lumbar coin stays pressed to the floor.

7. Take a deep, long sigh out as the arms float behind the head.

**REPETITIONS:** One set of ten.

**BREATHING:** As you contract forward, raising the legs into the air, breathe in to raise the arms from mid-thigh level to the vertical position. Ocean breathe out to take the arms behind the head and complete the circle to the hips, and breathe in to return to the rest position.

*Notes*

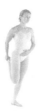

# Single Leg Circles 1

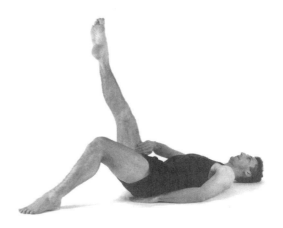

**PREREQUISITES:** The Start Stretches (Exercises 3 through 6a).

**PURPOSE:** To isolate the adductor muscle and mobilize the hip joint.

### EXERCISE DESCRIPTION:

*Starting Position:* Lie on the floor with both knees bent, thighs at a forty-five degree angle to the floor, feet flat on the floor. Decompress the spine. Place the hands on the floor, palms down, elbows slightly bent, with thumb and index finger just touching the buttock on each side. Engage the B-Line. Raise the right leg toward the ceiling, with the foot pointed, and turn out the leg. Press the left buttock against the thumb to stabilize the left side of the torso, and press the fingers of the right hand against the right adductor muscle, close to the groin, to connect the muscle.

a) Now make an inward circle with the right leg. Start by ocean breathing out to lower the leg, allowing the abdominals to lengthen. Extend through the toes as if you were drawing a circle on the ceiling with them. (The circle is actually a D shape, with a straight line down the middle to start.) Keep the other hip pressed into the mat.

b) Breathe in to circle the leg outward and raise it back up to the vertical position, maintaining the B-Line Core.

### KEY POINTS:

1. Do not allow the buttock of the resting leg to lift off the thumb at all.

2. Feel the inner thigh (adductor) muscle making the circle by pressing against the fingers to establish the connection. (Eventually, you can remove the fingers.)

3. Keep the circle high and small to start.

4. Do not push the supporting leg into the ground.

5. Press the imaginary sacrum coin onto the floor.

**REPETITIONS:** Complete six circles in one direction, then change legs. Repeat the circles in the other direction.

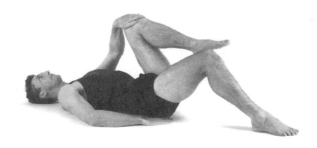

## Easier Variation: Knee Stirs

If this exercise is too difficult to perform for more than four repetitions, then try the following: Instead of extending a straight leg to the ceiling, bend the knee and place the hand on the kneecap. Make a circle away from the body only as far as the extension of the arm will allow. Imagine you are stirring a pot with the thigh bone. Gradually extend the foot into the air, keeping the hand on the knee until the leg is almost fully extended.

# Side to Side

**PREREQUISITES:** Warm-up stretches, and no major back problems.

**PURPOSE:** To strengthen the obliques while in an elongated position. To provide abdominal support for the back while in rotation.

### EXERCISE DESCRIPTION:

*Starting Position:* Lie on your back and draw the knees toward the chest. Take the knees just past the vertical (they will be directly above the lower ribs). Decompress the spine. Squeeze a thin pad between the knees. Keep the feet pointed and raised slightly higher than the knees. Extend your arms on the floor at shoulder level with the palms up.

a) Over to the side: Engage the B-Line Core and ocean breathe out to take both knees over to the right side, but only halfway to the floor. Keep the opposite shoulder blade on the floor at all times. Start the movement by peeling the right hip off the floor, keeping the knees level with each other and in line with the navel.

b) Return to center: Do not press your right arm against the floor to assist the body to return to the center. First engage the B-Line Core more firmly, and then breathe in to slowly roll the left side of the rib cage to the floor, imprinting the side of the body onto the floor from the shoulder blade to the hip. To begin rolling the spine to the floor, flatten the rib cage first and keep the knees in line with the ribs.

c) Without stopping, ocean breathe out to flow the movement to the left side.

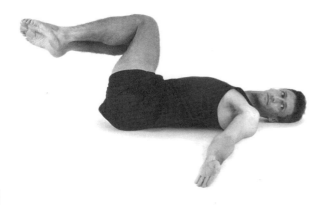

### KEY POINTS:

1. Press the knees together. Keep the feet slightly higher than the knees at all times.

2. Keep the shoulder blades pressed to the floor. Try not to move them.

3. When comfortable with the movement, turn the head in the opposite direction from the knees to rotate throughout the length of the spine.

4. The exercise should be felt in the abdominals only, never in the back.

5. When taking the legs over to the side, make sure to avoid twisting at the hips.

6. Both knees must move together to prevent the lower back from twisting.

7. When you return to the center, imprint the spine from the shoulder blade and then down the length of the spine to the hip.

**REPETITIONS:** Six to ten repetitions on each side.

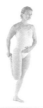

# Stomach Stretch

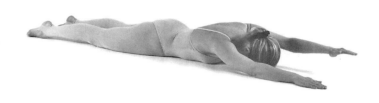

**PREREQUISITE:** The Hundreds: Basic (Exercise 18).

**PURPOSE:** To strengthen the abdominals in elongation, and to strengthen the back.

### EXERCISE DESCRIPTION:

*Starting Position:* Lie on the floor on your stomach (prone) with your arms stretched above the head, legs extended and hip distance apart, toes pointed. Rest your forehead on the ground or on a cushion to keep the neck in line with the upper back. Place a towel between the ribs and the hips if there is any pressure in the lower back.

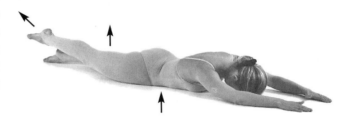

a) Engage the B-Line Core and scoop the abdominals to support the lower back. Ocean breathe out to extend the left arm two inches off the ground. Imagine that someone is holding your wrist and lengthening the limb out of the socket, while keeping the shoulders level (do not hunch the shoulders).

b) Breathe in to continue to extend the arm, lowering it to lightly touch the floor, and scooping the B-Line Core even more.

c) Ocean breathe out to extend the other arm.

### KEY POINTS:

1. Keep the B-Line Core so that a ruler could easily slide between the mat and your stomach at all times.

2. Lengthen through the crown of the head, and keep the shoulder blades pressed into the pocket.

3. If the back begins to take over, stop.

4. Attempt one more repetition each day to increase the abdominal work.

**REPETITIONS:** One set of ten alternating lifts.

**BASIC/INTERMEDIATE VARIATION:** Alternating Leg Lifts.

Follow the same procedure as in the preceding exercise, but this time use the legs instead of the arms.

### Notes

.......................................................

.......................................................

.......................................................

.......................................................

.......................................................

.......................................................

# The Perfect Abdominal Curl (PAC)

**PREREQUISITES**: The Start Stretches (Exercises 3 through 6a).

**PURPOSE**: To provide basic abdominal strength for all exercises.

### EXERCISE DESCRIPTION:

*Starting Position:* Lie on your back on the floor, with the knees together and bent at ninety degrees or more so the feet are placed on the floor approximately twenty-four inches from the buttocks. Decompress the spine. The entire back must be flat, in the Stable Spine position. Place your hands where they are most comfortable, either crossing the wrists behind the head so the hands are on the opposite shoulders to support the neck, or with fingers and thumbs interlocked behind the head and elbows wide open (photo), or with the arms crossed on the chest.

a) Engage the B-Line. Ocean breathe out to draw the ribs as close as possible to the hips, keeping them in a horizontal plane, until the shoulder blades come off the ground. Scoop the abdominals (imagine a greyhound's stomach).

b) Breathe in to slowly release the abdominals 10 percent; or allow the torso to lower so that the shoulder blades almost touch the floor, whichever creates the larger movement. Keep the eyes on the knees.

Without stopping, repeat ten times.

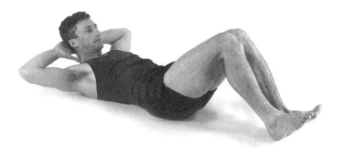

### KEY POINTS:

1. If the hands are behind the head, keep the elbows wide open. The arms are there to support the head, not to pull it forward.

2. Keep the chin off the chest and the eyes focused on the knees.

3. Imagine using the area between the ribs and the hips as a bellows that you close on the breath out and partially release on the breath in.

4. Contract forward without the ribs lifting above the level of the hips, as this can bunch the abdominals out.

5. Contract the abdominals to lift the head, neck, and shoulders, not the other way around.

6. Move smoothly, without using momentum or any jerky movements.

7. If the back arches, place the feet on a chair with the knees above the lower ribs.

**REPETITIONS**: Up to three sets of ten to twelve repetitions.

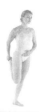

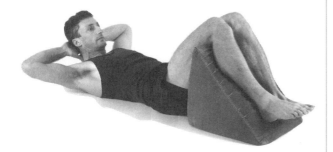

**VARIATIONS FOR GREATER
ABDOMINAL CONNECTION:**

1. Flex the feet so that you are lightly balancing on the heels.

2. Place the legs over high cushions so that
   when they are relaxed, the thighs do not
   flop open and the heels do not touch the
   ground. This position greatly reduces the
   connection of the front of the thighs
   (quadriceps) and the inner thighs (adductors). It also works the B-Line more specifically. Keep the thighs relaxed during the
   entire set.

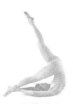

# Ankle Weights: Outer Thigh (Abductor)

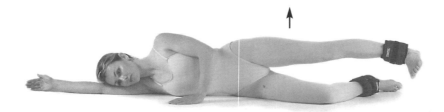

**PREREQUISITE:** None.

**PURPOSE:** To strengthen and tone the hip by working the outer hip and the back of the thighs. To stabilize the pelvis.

### EXERCISE DESCRIPTION:

This exercise may be done with any of the following:

- No ankle weights (the weight of the leg may be sufficient to begin)

- A two-pound weight on each leg

- A four- or five-pound weight on each leg (advanced and men only)

*Starting Position:* Lie on your right side with your body in a straight line. As in all routines done lying on the side, you should lie with your back against a wall to ensure correct spinal posture. Do not lean against the wall—just use it as a guide to maintain a straight back. Place the right arm under the head, extended in a line with the body, with the palm facing upward. Bend the right leg (bottom/supporting leg) as much as forty-five degrees, with the foot remaining in line with the body. Keeping the left leg straight, bring it six inches forward in order to help keep the back flat. Flex the left foot and raise the leg off the ground six inches.

The following are important for the perfect execution of the exercise:

a) Press the left hip away from the left rib with the left hand so that the left hip sits on top of the right hip. The hips are now aligned vertically. Engage the B-Line Core. Imagine that the weight is on the top of the thigh, about six inches from the hip joint.

b) Ocean breathe out to lengthen through the heel, raising the leg approximately six to twelve inches maximum above the height of the hip. You should feel the outer thigh working strongly.

c) Breathing in, lower the leg to just below hip level before repeating. Do not rest the leg on the floor.

### KEY POINTS:

1. Keep the hips aligned. An alternative to pressing the top hip away is to place the left hand, palm up, between the right side of the waist and the floor, closer to the hip. Now create a gap between the palm of the hand and the waist, without hunching the shoulder. As the leg lifts, attempt to increase the size of this gap. If the waist touches the hand every time the leg is raised, the leg is being raised too high, causing the hip to move.

2. Maintain the B-Line Core.

3. If the back tends to arch, tuck the pelvis so that the back is touching, but not pressing against, the wall.

4. Keep the top shoulder blade drawn into the pocket.

5. Lengthen through the heel at all times.

**REPETITIONS:** Ten to twenty on each leg.

**INCREASE THE CHALLENGE:** Bend the knee of the working leg so that it is "unlocked" for all the repetitions.

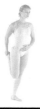

# Ankle Weights: Inner Thigh (Adductor)

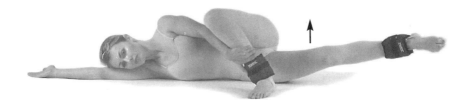

**PREREQUISITE:** None.

**PURPOSE:** To strengthen, while lengthening, the inner thigh.

### EXERCISE DESCRIPTION:

*Starting Position:* Lie on your right side with the right arm extended under the head, palm up, and the left hand relaxed on the floor. Place a high cushion next to the hip against the abdomen. Bend the left leg and rest it on top of the cushion. (If you don't have a cushion, place the left leg as illustrated in the photo.) Draw the right leg forward so the foot is twelve inches away from the wall behind you. Keep the right knee straight and facing forward and keep the foot pointed.

a) Imagine that the weight is sitting high on the inner right thigh, between the knee and the groin. Engage the B-Line Core, and ocean breathe out to raise the right inner thigh as high as possible without moving any other part of the body.

b) Still lengthening through the toe, breathe in to lower the leg about 90 percent before repeating the lift. Do not rest between repetitions.

### KEY POINTS:

1. Do not place any pressure on the cushion to lift the lower leg.

2. Engage the B-Line Core during the lifting and lowering of the leg.

3. Keep the bottom leg in front of the body.

4. If the bottom hip is uncomfortable, lie on a cushion.

**REPETITIONS:** One set of ten to twenty repetitions.

**INCREASE THE CHALLENGE:** Do one or both of the following:

1. Bend the knee of the working leg slightly, continuing to lengthen through the foot.

2. Turn out the lower (working) leg from the inner thigh, without moving the hips from their vertical position.

### Notes

.................................................................

.................................................................

.................................................................

.................................................................

# Ankle Weights: Outer Thigh Flexion (Abductor)

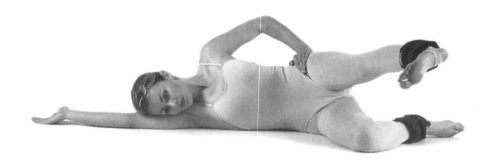

**PREREQUISITE:** Ankle Weights: Outer Thigh (Exercise 26-1).

**PURPOSE:** To strengthen the outer thigh when the leg is at a right angle to the body.

### EXERCISE DESCRIPTION:

This exercise may be done with any of the following:

- No ankle weights (the weight of the leg may be sufficient to begin)

- A two-pound weight on each leg

- A four- or five-pound weight on each leg (advanced and men only)

*Starting Position:* Lie on your right side with your back against a wall to ensure correct spinal posture. Do not lean against the wall—just use it as a guide to maintain a straight back. Place the right arm under the head, extended in a line with the body, with the palm facing upward. Bend the right leg to as much as forty-five degrees, keeping the foot in line with the body. Flex the left foot and raise the leg off the ground six inches.

a) Engage the B-Line and take the left leg as far forward as possible, at hip level, so that the top knee is directly above the bent knee. (If the top leg can go farther forward than the bottom leg and you feel unbal-anced, bend the bottom leg more so the knees remain vertically aligned with each other.) Ocean breathe out to lift the outer thigh so that the foot rises as much as six inches higher than the level of the hip. Do not lift from the foot.

b) Breathe in to lower the left leg just below the height of the hip. Repeat.

### KEY POINTS:

1. Keep the top hip aligned with the bottom one.

2. Press the left hip away from the left rib with the left hand so that it sits on top of the right hip. The hips are now aligned vertically.

3. This exercise is a challenge! Do not overdo it.

**REPETITIONS:** Ten to twenty on each side.

### INCREASE THE CHALLENGE:

1. Unlock the top knee.

2. Turn the working leg in toward the floor from the thigh without moving the hip.

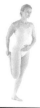

# Back of the Thigh: Hamstring/Buttocks

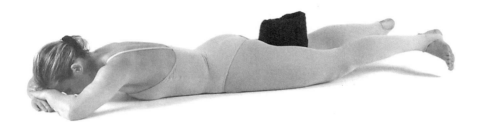

**PREREQUISITES:** Ankle Weights (Exercises 26-1 through 26-3).

**PURPOSE:** To strengthen the hamstring and tone and tighten the buttocks.

### EXERCISE DESCRIPTION:

*Starting Position:* Lie prone (on the stomach) with a flat cushion under the abdominals (between the ribs and the hips) and the forehead resting on the hands. The legs are extended and turned out, with the feet flexed. Place a thick pad between the legs and tightly into the crotch.

a) Engage the B-Line and ocean breathe out to raise the legs two inches and squeeze the pad. Try to touch the backs of your knees together. Keep the abdominals drawn up away from the cushion. Do not allow the hips to lift off the floor.

b) Breathe in to release 10 percent before repeating.

### KEY POINTS:

1. Keep the B-Line Core engaged to support the lower back.

2. Keep the shoulder blades drawn into the pocket.

3. To avoid arching the back, do not raise the legs higher than two inches

4. If the knees do touch, place a thicker pad in the groin.

**REPETITIONS:** Two sets of ten to twenty repetitions.

*Notes*

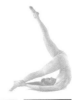

# Arm Weights: Position for All Supine Routines

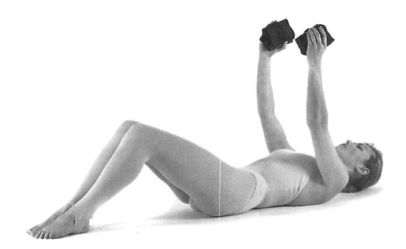

**PREREQUISITE:** None.

**PURPOSE:** To strengthen and mobilize the arms, chest, back, and neck.

**EXERCISE DESCRIPTION:** Base the amount of the weights you use on your strength. You can use heavier weights for Exercise 28-2, as no rotation of the joint is involved. If you do this exercise at home, you can use cans of beans in place of weights. All of these arm-weight exercises are done lying on the back (supine).

### KEY POINTS:

1. Lie on the floor or on a narrow bench, knees bent at a forty-five-degree angle.

2. Decompress the spine and maintain the B-Line Core and Stable Spine.

3. Keep the fingers extended to obtain maximum elongation from the shoulder joint.

4. Keep the arms positioned vertically above the chest, not above the face.

5. "Unlock" the elbows, but continue to elongate through the arm and out of the extended fingers.

6. Keep the neck long and the shoulder blades drawn into the pocket.

7. If the neck is arched, or if there is a large gap between the back of the neck and the bench or floor, place a cushion under the head for more comfort.

8. Imagine that the weight is near the top of the arm, about six inches from the shoulder. This makes it easier to lift the weight and to connect the upper arm muscles.

9. On the breath out, flatten the ribs to the floor to keep the thoracic spine stable.

10. If you have any "clicking" or strain in the shoulder joints, reduce the range of the movement.

11. Maintain the B-Line Core at all times.

*Notes*

.......................................................

.......................................................

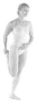

# Opening Arms

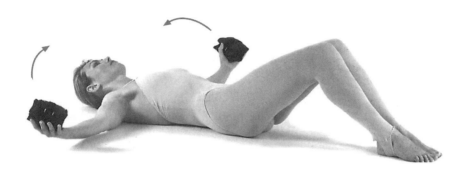

**PREREQUISITE AND PURPOSE:** Same as for Exercise 28-1.

**EXERCISE DESCRIPTION:**

a) Imagine that a huge beach ball is being pumped up between your arms and, breathing in, resist as the arms are pressed open to the sides.

b) Ocean breathe out to squeeze the air out of the beach ball on the upward movement. Feel the chest muscles (pectoral muscles) doing the work to raise the arms to the ceiling (imagine that a pencil is lying on your breastbone and you are trying to squeeze it with your chest muscles). Alternatively, get a friend to gently press against the pectoral muscles as you press against their fingers when closing.

**KEY POINTS:** Same as for Exercise 28-1.

**REPETITIONS:** One set of up to twenty repetitions.

*Notes*

.........................................................

.........................................................

.........................................................

.........................................................

.........................................................

.........................................................

.........................................................

.........................................................

.........................................................

# Alternating Arms

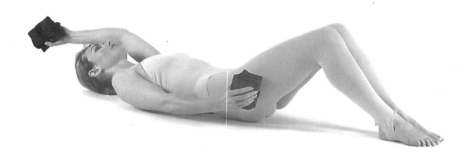

**PREREQUISITE AND PURPOSE:** Same as for Exercise 28-1.

### EXERCISE DESCRIPTION:

a) Ocean breathe out to extend the right arm down toward your right foot; at the same time extend the left arm to your left ear and to a point above your head, flattening the rib cage.

Do not hunch the left shoulder. Keep a gap between the left arm and the left ear. Only lower the weight 90 percent. If the left arm does not extend toward the level of the ear without the rib cage lifting, slowly release the left chest muscle.

b) Before returning to the upright position, engage the B-Line Core more firmly, flatten the rib cage, and breathe in to lift the arms to the ceiling. Lengthen the left arm by engaging the muscles in the back of the upper arm (the triceps). To connect this muscle and avoid shoulder strain, imagine squashing an orange under the armpit, or get a friend to gently apply pressure halfway between the elbow and the shoulder, and press against this.

If the left shoulder is raised slightly toward the ear, press it toward the hip before raising the arm to the ceiling. You should then get a better connection both above and below the shoulder joint (the latissimus dorsi will connect).

c) Raise both arms to the starting position and, without stopping in the vertical position, alternate the movement.

**KEY POINTS:** Same as for Exercise 28-1.

**REPETITIONS:** One set of ten on each side, alternating sides.

*Notes*

.................................................

.................................................

.................................................

.................................................

.................................................

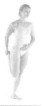

# Double Overhead Arms

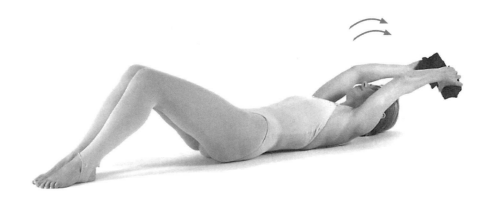

**PREREQUISITE AND PURPOSE:** Same as for Exercise 28-1.

**EXERCISE DESCRIPTION:**

*Starting Position:* Lightly touch the fingertips (or knuckles) of each hand together above the chest with the elbows bent slightly outward.

a) Engage the B-Line Core and ocean breathe out to extend both arms above the head to a point where the ribs do not lift, the back does not arch, and the shoulders do not hunch.

b) Do not rest the arms. Flatten the ribs to the floor, and press the shoulder blades toward the pocket.

c) Breathe in to float the arms back up to the ceiling. Imagine squashing oranges under the armpits to connect the back of the upper arms and the latissimus dorsi. Repeat without stopping.

**KEY POINTS:** Same as for Exercise 28-1.

**REPETITIONS:** One set of ten.

*Notes*

...................................................
...................................................
...................................................
...................................................
...................................................
...................................................
...................................................
...................................................
...................................................
...................................................

# Arm Circles

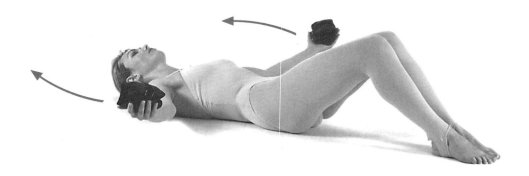

**PREREQUISITE AND PURPOSE:** Same as for Exercise 28-1.

### EXERCISE DESCRIPTION:

a) Engage the B-Line Core and breathe in to extend both hands down toward the heels, palms facing each other. If you're on a bench, do not allow the arms to go below bench level.

b) Turn the palms up to the ceiling and ocean breathe out to extend the arms out to the sides and around toward the head. Keep the arms just above bench or floor level, and move them until they reach as close to the ears as is comfortable.

c) At this point, keep moving, turning the palms to face inward, and breathe in to extend the arms to the ceiling and continue down toward the feet. If the shoulder joints are tight, you may make the circle smaller.

Remember to squeeze the imaginary oranges under the armpits when raising the arms from above the head to the ceiling and lowering them to the feet. Avoid bending the elbows any farther than the "unlocked" position for the entire routine.

**KEY POINTS:** Same as for Exercise 28-1.

**REPETITIONS:** One set of ten in one direction, then one set of ten in the other direction, that is, first lowering the arms back behind the head. Always start the routine by circling toward the heels first (inward circle).

*Notes*

.............................................................

.............................................................

.............................................................

.............................................................

.............................................................

.............................................................

.............................................................

.............................................................

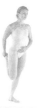

# Arm Swings: Alternating

**PREREQUISITE:** None.

**PURPOSE:** To mobilize the shoulder joints, stretch and open the chest (pectorals), and improve thoracic and cervical posture.

### EXERCISE DESCRIPTION:

*Starting Position:* Stand upright on the tripods of the feet, sideways to a mirror, feet placed hip distance apart.

a) Engage the B-Line Core and raise the arms in front of the torso to shoulder level, with the right palm down and the left palm up. Lengthen through the fingertips.

b) Ocean breathe out to extend the right arm to the ceiling and the left arm to the floor so both palms are facing forward. Do not hunch the right shoulder. Lengthen through the crown of the head. Flatten the ribs to an imaginary wall behind you on the breath out. This will stabilize the thoracic area and help stretch the chest muscles.

c) Continue to take the arms past the (vertical) line of the body. Look in the mirror to ensure that the back does not arch excessively. Imagine that you are standing against a wall that follows the natural curve of your spine, and that the gap between the wall and the lower back cannot increase. Hold the B-Line Core as firmly as possible.

d) Breathe in to lengthen the arms forward to the shoulder-level position. Now rotate the arms and hands so the right palm is up and the left palm is down, and breathe out to continue moving the arms, right arm toward the floor and left arm to the ceiling.

### KEY POINTS:

1. Maintain the tripod position and the B-Line Core.

2. Keep the ribs as flat as possible against the imaginary wall behind you to prevent them from protruding forward and arching the back. Lengthen through the fingertips.

3. Keep the neck long and upright, so it does not crane forward as the arms stretch past the vertical line.

4. Keep the shoulder blades drawn into the pocket.

**REPETITIONS:** One set of ten repetitions on each side, alternating sides.

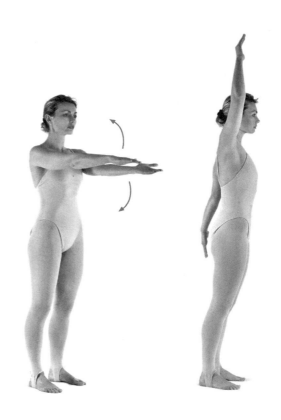

# Arm Swings: Chest Expansion

**PREREQUISITE AND PURPOSE:** Same as for Exercise 29-1.

**EXERCISE DESCRIPTION:**

The extended arms start with the hands at navel level, palms facing up to the ceiling.

a) Ocean breathe out to open the arms to a forty-five-degree angle and back behind the head at head level. Feel the stretch across the chest.

b) Breathe in to return the arms to the starting position.

**KEY POINTS:**

1. Same as for Exercise 29-1.

2. Press the shoulder blades toward the pocket at all times.

3. Do not jut the chin out.

**REPETITIONS:** One set of ten repetitions.

*Notes*

. . . . . . . . . . . . . . . . . . . . . . . . . . . . . . . . . . . . . . .

. . . . . . . . . . . . . . . . . . . . . . . . . . . . . . . . . . . . . . .

. . . . . . . . . . . . . . . . . . . . . . . . . . . . . . . . . . . . . . .

. . . . . . . . . . . . . . . . . . . . . . . . . . . . . . . . . . . . . . .

. . . . . . . . . . . . . . . . . . . . . . . . . . . . . . . . . . . . . . .

. . . . . . . . . . . . . . . . . . . . . . . . . . . . . . . . . . . . . . .

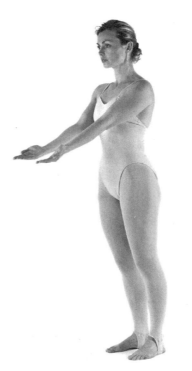

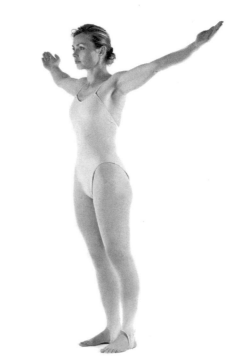

# The Pole

**PREREQUISITES:** Exercises 28-2 and 28-3.

**PURPOSE:** To open the chest fully, stretch the pectoral muscles, and improve rotation of the shoulder joints.

### EXERCISE DESCRIPTION:

*Starting Position:* Facing a mirror, engage the B-Line Core and hold on to a pole, broomstick, or Theraband at shoulder level, hands comfortably wide apart and palms down. Hold the pole with only the thumb and forefinger wrapped around it. The other fingers remain extended, in order to prevent torsion in the wrist joint and straining of the neck once the movement has started.

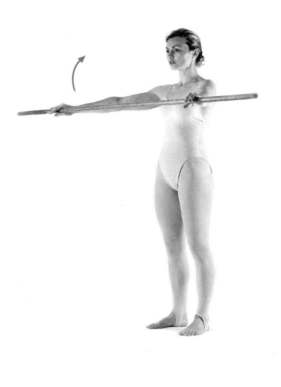

a) Imagine that your shoulders are the radius of a circle. Lengthening your arms while holding the pole in front of you, breathe in to raise the pole toward the ceiling without hunching the shoulders.

b) Ocean breathe out to lower the pole behind the shoulders and down toward the floor, lengthening through the arms the entire time. Do not bend the elbows. If they, or the shoulders or chest, are too tight, widen your hold on the pole. Lengthen the neck toward the ceiling. Do not jut the chin forward.

c) Hold the position with the pole behind your buttocks for the breath in. Engage the B-Line Core and ocean breathe out to once again press the pole behind the shoulders toward the far wall, up toward the ceiling, and forward to shoulder level.

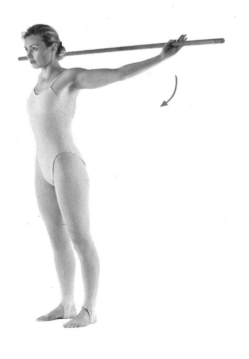

# The Pole *(cont'd.)*

### KEY POINTS:

1. Look in the mirror to ensure that the pole is always parallel to the floor.

2. Maintain the tripod position at all times; do not rock onto the toes or heels.

3. Do not crane the neck forward.

4. Ocean breathe out deeply to take the arms behind you at shoulder-blade level on the way up and down.

**REPETITIONS:** Ten repetitions (backward and forward is one repetition).

*Notes*

.................................................

.................................................

.................................................

.................................................

.................................................

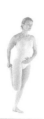

# 8

## THE INTERMEDIATE ROUTINE

Correctly
executed and
mastered to
the point of
subconscious
reaction, these
exercises will
reflect grace and
balance in your
routine activities.

— J. PILATES

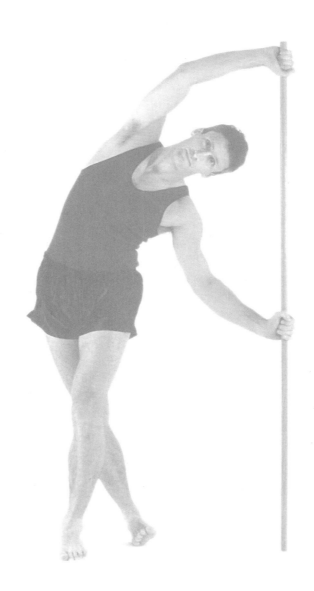

# The Hundreds: Alternating Legs

**PREREQUISITE:** The Hundreds: Basic (Exercise 18).

**PURPOSE:** To work each side of the abdominals separately.

### EXERCISE DESCRIPTION:

*Starting Position:* Lie on your back and decompress your spine. Draw the legs to the chest and hold on to the knees. Rest your head on the floor and keep your neck long. Contract forward (head and shoulders forward, eyes on the knees, ribs drawn as close as possible toward the hips). Extend the legs vertically into the air, feet pointed, legs turned out.

a) Extend the arms past the hips, palms facing inward, lengthening through the fingertips and keeping the hands several inches off the floor. Press the shoulder blades toward the hips. Engage the B-Line and ocean breathe out to flex the right foot and lower the right leg as close to the floor as you can while keeping the imaginary lumbar coin pressed against the floor. Leave the left leg in the air, drawing it slightly closer to the chest. This is the leg that makes the abdominals work harder!

b) Engage the B-Line more firmly and breathe in to raise the right leg back to the vertical position. Change legs.

### KEY POINTS:

1. As the leg lowers, draw the ribs even closer to the hips to counteract any drop of the shoulders.

2. Keep the shoulder blades raised off the floor when lifting the leg back to the vertical position.

3. Ensure that the vertical leg is totally straight and turned out, with the foot flexed.

4. Keep the eyes on the knees, and breathe into the armpits.

5. Do not lower the leg too low; keep the lumbar coin pressed down.

6. Lengthen the abdominals and allow the thigh muscles to stretch to achieve a controlled lowering of the leg—imagine that the hip joint is opening like a hinge.

**REPETITIONS:** Five to ten repetitions for each leg.

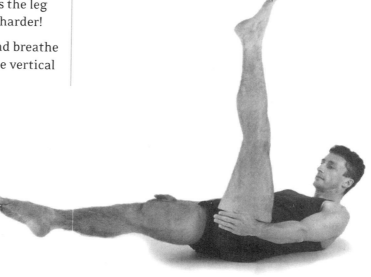

# Coordination

**PREREQUISITE:** The Hundreds: Basic (Exercise 18).

**PURPOSE:** To coordinate the arms and legs with the breath. To work the adductors, shoulders, upper back, and abdominals.

### EXERCISE DESCRIPTION:

*Starting Position:* Lie on your back with your knees drawn comfortably to your chest, tailbone on the mat, hands on the knees, and elbows bent.

a) Engage the B-Line and ocean breathe out to contract forward, extending the arms past the hips, lengthening through the finger-tips, and extending the legs forward as low as you can while still keeping the imaginary lumbar coin pressed into the mat (legs parallel, toes softly pointed).

b) Hold the breath to rapidly open and close the legs once, attempting to engage the inner thighs for the movement. (Open the legs just wider than shoulder distance.)

c) Breathe in to return to the starting position (bending the knees to the chest) for half a second before repeating.

### KEY POINTS:

1. Stretch through the toes as far as you can, even when opening and closing the legs.

2. When returning to the starting position, draw the knees to the chest (rather than dropping the feet to the bottom).

3. Keep the B-Line engaged even when returning to the starting position.

4. Keep the abdominals "scooped" until all repetitions are completed.

5. Squeeze the inner thighs together until the final repetition is complete.

6. Focus mentally on every movement of the arms, head, neck, shoulders, legs, and inner thighs, as well as on the breathing.

**REPETITIONS:** One set of ten.

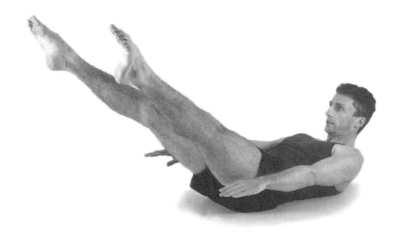

# The Roll-Up

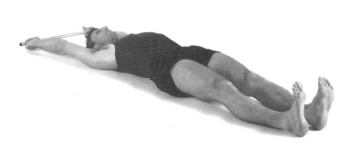
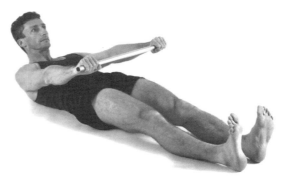

**PREREQUISITES:** The Start Stretches (Exercises 3 through 6a), The Perfect Abdominal Curl (Exercise 25).

**PURPOSE:** To strengthen the abdominals through the full range of movement while stretching the back.

### EXERCISE DESCRIPTION:

*Starting Position:* Hold on to a short pole (a small towel stretched between your hands will do). Lie on your back on a mat, arms above your head on the floor, elbows extended, legs straight, feet flexed, pressing through your heels, inner thighs squeezed together.

a) Engage the B-Line and take a long breath in to raise the (straight) arms toward the ceiling and then lower them to your thighs, flattening the ribs to the floor. Roll the chin to the chest at the same time.

b) Ocean breathe out to curl the shoulders forward and draw the ribs to the hips, rolling forward off the floor in a smooth movement. Continue to roll each vertebra off the mat, at the same time pressing your spine into the mat.

c) Once you're sitting up, reach forward as far as you can, lengthening your chest toward your knees and the crown of your head to-

ward your toes. Hold this position and take a deep breath into your back and armpits.

d) Still reaching the arms toward the feet and pressing through the heels, ocean breathe out to roll back down. Start by sinking into the hips, looking into the groin and imprinting the spine into the mat one vertebra at a time until the arms are above the head on the floor. Maintain your B-Line at all times.

### KEY POINTS:

1. Exhale 75 percent of your breath during the first 25 percent of the movement or when the head and shoulders are lifting off the floor.

2. On the return movement, exhale 75 percent of the breath during the first 25 percent of the movement after sinking into the hips. If the lungs are too full of air, the back may move as a stiff block, rather than rolling.

3. Keep reaching forward on the way up as if someone were pulling the pole forward for you. On the way down, lean forward as if someone were trying to pull you to your toes. This has the effect of opening up the back. Keep the pole close to the thighs on the way up and down.

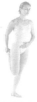

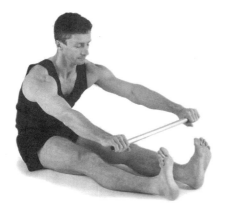

4. If the spine fails to roll smoothly all the way (up or down), bend the knees.

5. If, on the roll up, the torso lifts rather than rolls, bend the knees more or place light weights on your feet.

**REPETITIONS:** One set of ten repetitions.

**BREATHING REVIEW:** Ocean breathe out to roll up, breathe in to stretch forward, and ocean breathe out to roll down.

## THE PSOAS AND ITS EFFECT ON THE LOWER BACK

*The psoas (hip flexor) and its effect on the lower back during roll-ups or conventional sit-ups is greatly underestimated. The psoas attaches from the lower vertebrae of the spine, crosses in front of the hip, and attaches to the upper inside of the femur (the lesser trochanter). When you relax the abdominals between repetitions (even for a fraction of a second), or hold your breath during the exercise, the torso will lift off the floor and the hip flexors will engage at the same time, pulling the body up rather than rolling it up. This action is more apparent when the feet are hooked under a strap. It happens because the psoas grips, thereby controlling the movement, lifting the lower lumbar vertebrae, and slightly distending the abdominals. This action, in combination with weak abdominals, prevents the psoas from depressing, which would allow the spine to roll up. The result is a lift of the back.*

*Instead of completing ten "individual" movements, keep the abdominals and hip flexors connected (engaged) and try to perform ten continuous, flowing movements. Think of the set as one movement comprising ten continuous parts.*

*If the hip flexors are continuously engaged and the abdominals are in a strong B-Line (to assist in controlling the psoas) before the roll-up begins, the chances of a lurch are greatly minimized. Initially, the thighs may feel overworked. However, as the abdominals retain the engram (memory) of the rolling movement, they will supersede any hip flexor strain. When the feet are in a strap to assist in the roll-up, imagine that the strap is a thin thread of cotton and that any mild pull of the feet will snap the thread. Doing so will also help to partially disengage the psoas and to engage the abdominals more effectively.*

*The feet should remain flexed at all times. Placing them in a strap around the toes only engages the thighs even more. Instead, place the strap close to the ankles. Squeezing the inner thighs may also help slightly to alleviate some of the gripping of the thighs.*

# The Roll-Over

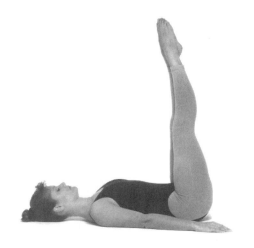

**PREREQUISITES:** Two sets of The Hundreds: Intermediate (Exercise 19-1) with low legs, and an absence of neck problems.

**PURPOSE:** To mobilize and massage the length of the spine and to open the spaces between the vertebrae while flexing the spine. This exercise is similar to the yoga plow.

**EXERCISE DESCRIPTION:**

*Starting Position:* Lie on your back on the floor and decompress the spine. The legs are vertical and the feet are pointed and turned out. Squeeze the backs of the knees toward each other, and place your hands by your sides, palms down. Engage the B-Line.

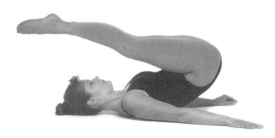

a) Ocean breathe out to draw the thighs toward the rib cage (still keeping the legs straight), folding from the hips, and continue rolling over smoothly. Elongate the legs, drawing your knees as close as you can toward your nose until the feet touch the floor behind your head, if possible. Keep your legs straight. Roll over onto the top of the shoulders, and no farther, lengthening the neck. Maintain the B-Line.

b) Breathe in to turn the legs parallel and open them to just past shoulder width apart. Flex the feet.

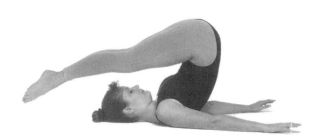

c) Ocean breathe out to roll the spine down one vertebra at a time, imprinting it back onto the mat until the legs have returned to the starting position (vertical). Lengthen through the fingers to relax the shoulders.

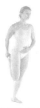

## KEY POINTS:

1. Imagine you have heavy weights around your ankles, and keep your knees stretched straight. This will keep the legs closer to the body and increase the stretch of the spine and hamstrings. Use light to medium ankle weights if this helps.

2. On the way back to the floor, graze your thighs along your chest, extending through the heels toward the wall above your head.

3. Move the legs over your head smoothly, without using momentum; use only the strength from your abdominals.

4. Keep the thighs close to your chest on the roll-over (draw the hips to the ribs) and on the roll down (lengthen the hips away from the ribs).

5. Concentrate on keeping the stomach scooped.

6. Keep the shoulders relaxed, lengthening through the fingers.

7. Do not roll onto the neck.

8. Obtain more stretch in the hamstrings and spine by flexing the feet with the legs parallel, anchoring the toes into the floor, and pressing into the heels. Keep off the neck.

9. "Lengthen" the abdominals on the roll down to prevent the neck from arching and the shoulders from lifting.

**REPETITIONS:** Five repetitions as just described and five in the reverse direction: Roll over with the legs apart, feet flexed and parallel. Roll down with the legs together and turned out, feet pointed.

*Notes*

# Single Leg Circles

**PREREQUISITE:** Single Leg Circles 1 (Exercise 22).

**PURPOSE:** To isolate the adductor muscle and to mobilize the hip joint.

### EXERCISE DESCRIPTION:

*Starting Position:* Lie on the floor with both legs bent, feet flat on the floor about two feet from the buttocks. Decompress the spine. Extend the arms out to the sides on the floor, palms up. Engage the B-Line Core. Raise the right leg toward the ceiling, point the foot, and turn out the leg. Press the left buttock into the mat.

a) Make an inward circle with the right leg. Start by ocean breathing out to take the leg down to the floor, allowing the abdominals to stretch, and keeping the imaginary lumbar coin pressed to the floor.

b) Breathe in to extend through the toes while making a large circle out to the far right; raise the leg to the vertical position and back to the center. Engage the B-Line Core at all times.

The circle is a rapid movement as the leg is lowered and extended to the side. It is a slower movement as the leg is raised and crosses the body. Eventually, at-tempt to make the circle as close to the floor as possible, keeping it the same distance from the floor even while you take it out to the side, without allowing the opposite hip to move at all.

### KEY POINTS:

1. Feel the inner thigh (adductor) muscle making the circle. Do this by placing the fingers against the inner thigh near the groin and pressing firmly.

2. Keep the circle high and small to start. Do not allow the leg to lower too far if doing so causes the lumbar coin to lift.

3. Keep the left (nonworking) foot in the tri-pod position. As an option, place the thumb of the left hand under the left buttock (left palm down); keep the buttock pressed against the thumb and keep the knee upright at all times.

4. Do not push the arms into the floor.

**REPETITIONS:** Six circles in one direction, then change legs. Repeat in the other direction.

**INCREASE THE CHALLENGE:** Extend the bent leg onto the floor, with the foot flexed and upright.

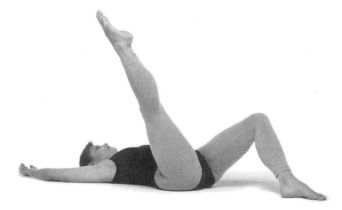
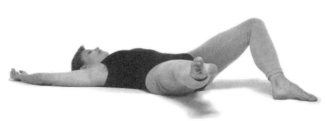

# Double Leg Stretch 2: Lowering and Raising

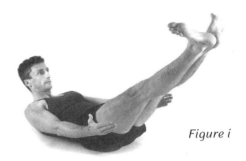

*Figure i*

**PREREQUISITES:** Preparation for the Hundreds (Exercise 17), Double Leg Stretch: Basic (Exercise 21), The Hundreds: Alternating Legs (Exercise 31), and Coordination (Exercise 32).

**PURPOSE:** To gain abdominal strength and control when moving the lower limbs, as well as to increase breathing control and shoulder mobility.

### EXERCISE DESCRIPTION:

*Starting Position:* Get into the starting position for the basic Double Leg Stretch (Exercise 21), and then extend the legs just past the vertical position, away from the body (Exercise 21, step a). Press the imaginary lumbar coin against the floor. Complete the arm circle (Exercise 21, steps b and c).

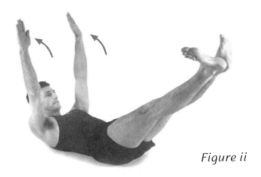

*Figure ii*

a)  Take a deep breath in to move the hands past the hips, bringing them even with the middle of the thigh. At the same time, raise the legs toward the ceiling.

b)  Ocean breathe out to lower the legs as low as you can, keeping the lumbar coin pressed into the floor, the feet flexed and turned out, and squeezing the inner thighs together (Figure i).

c)  Engage the B-Line more firmly and breathe in to raise the legs back to the near-vertical position, still squeezing the inner thighs together.

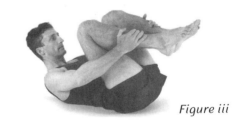

*Figure iii*

d)  Ocean breathe out to complete a second circle with the arms (Figure ii).

e)  Breathe in to return to the starting position (Figure iii).

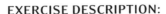

### KEY POINTS:

1.  When lowering the legs, press through the heels and squeeze the backs of the knees together.

2.  Keep the shoulder blades just off the floor at all times. It is important to prevent the head and shoulders from lowering as the legs lower. Allowing the head and shoulders to lower may arch the back, which may then strain when lifting the legs.

3.  You should feel as if the abdominals are flattening and lengthening to allow the legs to lower.

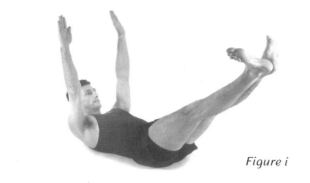

*Figure i*

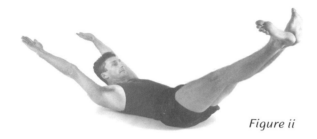

*Figure ii*

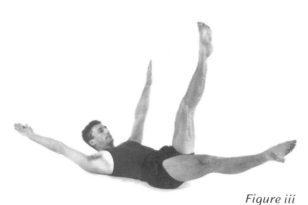

*Figure iii*

7. Always keep the lumbar coin pressed into the floor.

**REPETITIONS:** One set of ten, with half a second of rest between each repetition.

**BREATHING REVIEW:** Ocean breathe out to contract forward. Breathe in to move the arms to the vertical position. Ocean breathe out to move the arms around in a big circle. Breathe in to take the arms to mid-thigh level and the legs to the ceiling. Ocean breathe out to lower the legs. Breathe in to raise the legs. Ocean breathe out to complete the second full circle (optional). Breathe in to rest for half a second.

### INCREASE THE CHALLENGE

**PREREQUISITE:** Double Leg Stretch 2 (Exercise 36).

Follow all the instructions for the Double Leg Stretch, and then continue as described in the instructions that follow.

**ARMS TO CEILING:** After completing the first circle:

a) Breathe in to raise your arms and legs to the vertical position.

b) Ocean breathe out to lower the legs and continue as before (Figure i).

**ARMS TO EARS:** After completing the first circle:

a) Breathe in to raise your arms past the vertical position so that they are in line with your ears and to raise your legs toward the ceiling.

b) Ocean breathe out to lower the legs and continue as before (Figure ii).

**EXPANSION:** After completing the first circle:

a) Breathe in to raise the arms vertically.

b) Ocean breathe out to lower the right leg and extend the right arm to the right ear.

c) Breathe in to raise the leg and arm to vertical.

d) Ocean breathe out to repeat with the other arm and leg. Continue as before (Figure iii).

4. When raising the legs, engage the B-Line first, scoop the abdominals, and feel the hips drawing toward the rib cage. Feel as if the action of the abdominals contracting is what raises the legs into the air, rather than lifting from the thighs.

5. If the exercise is too challenging at first, return to the resting position after the legs have been raised—do not complete the second arm circle.

6. If, after several repetitions, the back begins to arch, keep the legs higher.

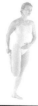

# Rolling Like a Ball

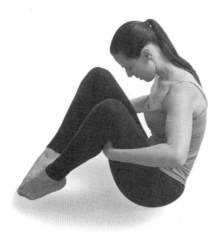
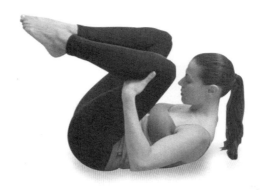

**PREREQUISITES:** The Roll-Up (Exercise 33), The Perfect Abdominal Curl (Exercise 25).

**PURPOSE:** To stretch and mobilize the spine.

### EXERCISE DESCRIPTION:

*Starting Position:* Sit on the floor on a mat with your heels drawn to your tailbone, forehead resting between your knees, which should be slightly apart. Your big toes should be touching. Hold on to your legs just behind your knees. Engage the B-Line.

a) Ocean breathe out to sink into your hips and round your back. Then breath in to roll smoothly onto your spine up to your shoulder blades (and no farther), keeping your heels to your tailbone and your nose to your knees.

b) Sharply ocean breathe out to pull your heels to your buttocks to initiate the movement back to the upright position. Balance on your tailbone with the toes lightly touching the floor.

### KEY POINTS:

1. Keep the heels close to the tailbone.

2. Roll only onto the shoulders, not onto the neck.

3. Sink into the hips to start the movement; this will help curl the tailbone to start the smooth roll. If you find that you roll to one side of the mat at first, this indicates that that side of your back is tighter than the other. This action will become less pronounced as you perform more sets and gain better control.

4. If you experience flat spots along the spine, or if the exercise is too challenging, start by lying on your back with your hands behind your knees, and attempt to roll up from the floor with a rocking movement. Bring the heels toward the buttocks to come up, and raise your feet toward the ceiling to roll back.

**REPETITIONS:** One set of ten rolls.

# Crisscross

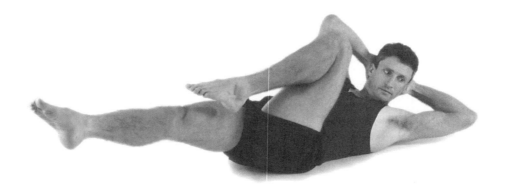

**PREREQUISITES:** The Perfect Abdominal Curl (Exercise 25), Single Leg Stretch (Exercise 20).

**PURPOSE:** To strengthen the obliques.

### EXERCISE DESCRIPTION:

In essence, this exercise combines the Perfect Abdominal Curl and the Single Leg Stretch.

*Starting Position:* Lying on the floor, decompress the spine. Contract forward with the fingers and thumbs interlocked behind the head and the elbows open. Engage the B-Line.

    a) Ocean breathe out to curl the body forward, drawing the right armpit toward the left knee, drawing the knee toward the left shoulder. Extend the right leg, turned out and with toes pointed, as low to the floor as possible, keeping the imaginary lumbar coin pressed to the floor. Scoop the stomach.

    b) Breathe in to change legs and release the torso until the shoulder blades almost touch the floor.

Repeat on the other side.

**KEY POINTS:**

1. Keep the shoulder blades off the floor at all times.

2. Keep the elbows wide open so there is no strain on the neck.

3. Turn the head and shoulders and look to the side wall for maximum rotation of the torso (where the eyes go, the body follows).

4. Keep the hips as still as possible so they don't sway from side to side.

5. Maintain the B-Line at all times. Be sure to extend the legs in line with the hip, not out to the sides.

6. Keep the chin off the chest.

**REPETITIONS:** One set of ten on each side.

**INCREASE THE CHALLENGE:** Think of turning and lifting forward while looking to the side wall. If you think of drawing the nipple to the knee this will create a greater rotation and contraction.

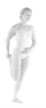

# Stomach Stretch: Alternating Arms and Legs

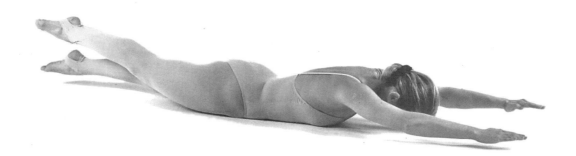

**PREREQUISITE:** Stomach Stretch (Exercise 24).

**PURPOSE:** To strengthen the back muscles.

### EXERCISE DESCRIPTION:

*Starting Position:* Lie on the stomach with the arms and legs extended, shoulder width apart. Place a small, flat cushion between the hips and the ribs to help support the B-Line Core. Rest the forehead on the floor or on a cushion. Point the toes and slightly turn out the legs.

a) Maintaining the B-Line Core, ocean breathe out to lift and lengthen the opposite arm and leg (right arm and left leg, or vice versa). Raise them less than two inches off the floor. Pinch the buttocks, but do not grip. At the same time, imagine that your abdominals are like a greyhound's stomach.

b) Keeping the buttocks pinched, breathe in to slowly lower the arm and leg and switch to the other arm and leg.

### KEY POINTS:

1. Maintain the B-Line Core to prevent the back from arching.

2. Allow the movement to flow smoothly.

3. Continue to "hold" the muscles of the arm and leg that stay in contact with the floor (i.e., don't allow them to fully rest).

4. Relax the neck, drawing the shoulder blades toward the hips. Lengthen through the tips of the fingers and toes.

5. If you feel any twinges in the back, open the legs wider. If it continues, stop the exercises.

6. If your head drops below the level of the shoulders, place the forehead on a higher cushion, so the neck is in line with the upper back.

**REPETITIONS:** Six to ten lifts on each side.

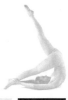

# Single Leg Kick

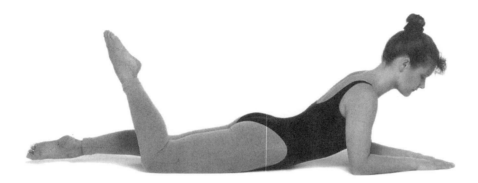

**PREREQUISITES:** The Hundreds: Intermediate (Exercise 19-1) and a strong back.

**PURPOSE:** To firm the hamstrings and buttocks, strengthen the abdominals in an elongated position, and stretch the front of the thighs.

### EXERCISE DESCRIPTION:

*Starting Position:* Lie on your stomach on the floor, legs extended, toes pointed.

a) Engage the B-Line Core and rise up onto your elbows, keeping them directly below your shoulders, palms down and pressed into the mat. Lengthen through the crown of the head without arching your neck. Keep the hips pressed into the mat and lift your chest as high as you can, stretching the abdominals, but maintaining the B-Line Core to support the back. Stretch through the toes, legs shoulder distance apart, pinch the buttocks firmly, and lift the feet just off the ground.

b) Ocean breathe out to rapidly kick your right foot to your buttock twice. On the second kick, lower the foot only halfway to the floor and then kick to the buttock with the foot flexed.

c) Point the foot and breathe in to lower the leg 90 percent.

d) Change legs.

### KEY POINTS:

1. If the hips lift off the floor and the back feels tight, extend the elbows farther in front of you, so that your back is longer.

2. Ensure the hipbones stay on the floor to keep the buttocks firm.

3. Keep the rib cage lengthened away from the hips.

4. Use a "percussion" breath out ("hah, hah") for each double kick.

5. If you feel the back starting to take any pressure, squeeze the B-Line Core more firmly.

6. Keep the shoulder blades drawn into the pocket and the neck long.

**REPETITIONS:** One set of five kicks on each leg, alternating legs.

**BREATHING REVIEW:** Double ocean breathe out on the double kick. Breathe in to lower the leg.

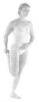

# Double Leg Kick

**PREREQUISITE:** Single Leg Kick (Exercise 40).

**PURPOSE:** To firm the buttocks and hamstrings, strengthen the back, and open the chest.

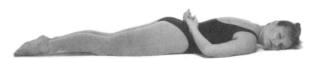

*Figure i*

### EXERCISE DESCRIPTION:

*Starting Position:* Lie on your stomach with your head turned to the right. Engage the B-Line Core. Keep the legs straight and shoulder distance apart, feet pointed. Hold one hand with the other, and place the hands in the small of the back (Figure i).

a) Double "percussion" breath out to rapidly kick both feet toward your buttocks twice (Figure ii).

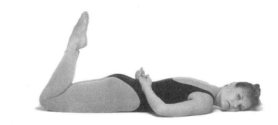

*Figure ii*

b) Breathe in to stretch the legs away from the body, raising the knees about six inches off the ground. At the same time, stretch your hands toward your feet, still holding them together, and lift your chest off the floor as high as possible without arching your neck. Look toward the wall in front of you (Figure iii).

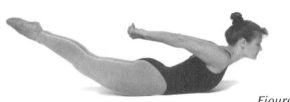

*Figure iii*

c) Breathe in to return to the starting position, turning your head to the other direction (to the left).

### KEY POINTS:

1. Press the shoulder blades into the pocket and keep the neck long.

2. As you lift the chest off the ground, squeeze the B-Line Core more firmly.

3. Squeeze the buttocks firmly throughout the routine.

4. Reduce the lift of the torso if you feel tightness in the shoulders, neck, or lower back.

5. Keep the legs wide open when raising the torso, to reduce pressure in the back.

**REPETITIONS:** One set of ten kicks, alternating the direction of the head each time.

**BREATHING REVIEW:** Double "percussion" breathe out to kick twice, breathe in to lift and lengthen, and ocean breathe out to lower the torso and repeat the kicks.

# Swan Dive 1

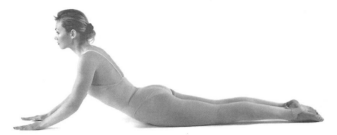

*Figure i*

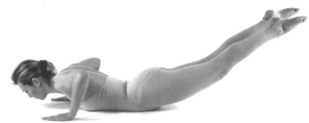

*Figure ii*

**PREREQUISITES:** Thigh Stretch 3: Kneeling (Exercise 13), The Perfect Abdominal Curl (Exercise 25), Stomach Stretch: Alternating Arms and Legs (Exercise 39).

**PURPOSE:** To strengthen the back and increase back control.

### EXERCISE DESCRIPTION:

*Starting Position:* Lie on the stomach in the push-up position, elbows on the ground and hands even with the top of the head, fingers forward. Lengthen through your toes with your legs in a comfortable position (shoulder distance apart). Engage the B-Line Core and keep the buttocks firm but not gripping.

a) Raise the legs slightly off the ground and take a deep breath in to straighten your arms as you raise your chest off the mat, letting your thighs stay in contact with the mat. Lengthen the crown of the head high without feeling any pressure along the spine (Figure i). Lock your body into this position.

b) Ocean breathe out to bend the elbows and rock forward slowly. The legs should rise into the air (thighs off the ground), lifting

from the hamstrings. Reaching the toes toward the ceiling, roll as far forward onto your breastbone as possible, eyes facing the floor (Figure ii).

c) Immediately rock back into the straight-arm position (Figure i).

### KEY POINTS:

1. If this movement is uncomfortable on the pubic bone, place a cushion under the hips. Keep the movement smooth at all times, with rhythmic breathing.

2. To rise up, focus on lifting the shoulder blades toward the ceiling.

3. To rock forward, focus on lifting the hamstrings toward the ceiling.

4. Keep lengthening through the crown of the head and through the point of the toes.

5. Keep the shoulder blades drawn into the pocket at all times.

6. Maintain the B-Line Core.

**REPETITIONS:** Three to eight repetitions.

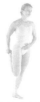

# Swan Dive 2

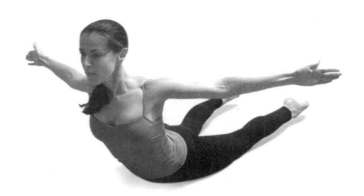

The exercise is the same as that in Exercise 42-1.

a) After straightening the arms to lift the torso, in a rapid movement raise the arms out to the sides in line with the shoulders and rock forward.

b) Keeping the arms at shoulder level, breathe in to "throw" the arms back to rock up.

c) Ocean breathe out to rock as far forward onto your breastbone as possible, keeping your head up, before breathing in to rock back as high as you can.

Continue rocking, keeping the movement as smooth as possible. Maintain the B-Line Core at all times.

Complete three to eight repetitions. Follow all the other instructions for Exercise 42-1.

**Notes**

# Swimming

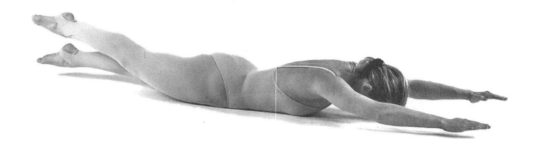

**PREREQUISITES:** Stomach Stretch: Alternating Arms and Legs (Exercise 39).

**PURPOSE:** To strengthen the back muscles and mobilize the hips and shoulders.

### EXERCISE DESCRIPTION:

*Starting Position:* Lie on the floor on your stomach, with your arms and legs extended, feet shoulder distance apart.

a) Engage the B-Line Core, lightly tighten the buttocks, and lift the arms, chest, and legs two inches off the floor. Lengthen through the tips of the fingers and toes, keeping the shoulders and pelvis square. Draw the shoulder blades into the pocket.

b) From this position, raise the right arm and left leg four inches higher. Take a long ocean breath out to quickly alternate lowering and lifting the arms and legs five times. (Right leg is lifted as left arm is lifted, and vice versa.)

c) Now breathe in for five beats (pumps) of the arms and legs. Continue for ten breaths in and out.

**KEY POINTS:**

1. Maintain the B-Line Core.

2. Keep the shoulders relaxed and the shoulder blades drawn into the pocket.

3. Extend the arms and legs through the fingertips and toes.

4. Imagine lifting and beating the legs from the hamstrings and the arms from the triceps.

5. Keep the legs at a height where the abdominals are pulled away from the floor, to prevent the back from taking over.

6. If this is too challenging, do the legs only with the head resting on the hands.

**REPETITIONS:** One set of ten breaths in and out.

*Notes*

...........................................................

...........................................................

...........................................................

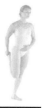

# Spine Rotation

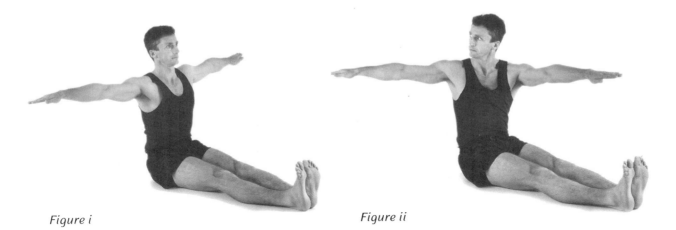

*Figure i*        *Figure ii*

**PREREQUISITES:** The Start Stretches (Exercises 3 through 6a).

**PURPOSE:** To provide mobility in the spine in rotation, and to focus on lifting out of the hips.

### EXERCISE DESCRIPTION:

*Starting Position:* On a mat, sit upright on your sitz bones with your legs extended straight in front of you. Flex your feet as you press through your heels, at the same time keeping your heels together. Squeeze the inner thighs together. Grow tall out of your spine as if sliding up a pole. Raise your arms out to the sides at shoulder height, palms down, stretching through the fingertips; lift the ribs away from the hips, and stretch the crown of your head to the ceiling (Figure i).

a) Engage the B-Line Core and ocean breathe out to rotate the torso toward the right as far as you can, sliding up the pole. Initiate the movement from the rib cage; imagine closing the ribs to rotate, maintaining an erect posture (Figure ii).

b) When you have rotated as far as you can, hold the position for half a second (keeping the ribs flat and the posture erect), and ocean breathe out again to rotate a little farther, this time drawing the right shoulder blade as far back as possible.

c) Take a deep breath in to return to the starting position, and, without stopping at the center, smoothly flow into a rotation in the other direction.

### KEY POINTS:

1. Keep lifted out of the hips.

2. Keep the shoulder blades pressed into the pocket at all times.

3. Turn the head along with the shoulders, and feel the movement loosening the rib cage area.

4. Keep the hips square by pressing through the right heel when turning to the right and through the left heel when turning to the left.

5. Do only the number of repetitions that is comfortable for the neck and shoulders.

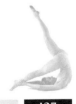

# Spine Rotation *(cont'd.)*

6. Perform the movement slowly and without much rotation at first; as you warm up go faster, increasing the rotation each time.

7. If the neck feels tight, either:

    i) interlock the fingers behind the head, keeping the elbows wide open; or

    ii) cross the hands in front of the chest and place them on the shoulders.

8. Perform only one rotation (that is, skip the extra breath out) if doing so is more comfortable.

9. Look over your shoulder, not to the floor.

10. Bend the knees if you can't sit tall.

11. Keep constantly sliding up the pole with the B-Line Core engaged.

**REPETITIONS:** Ten full rotations.

*Notes*

...................................................

...................................................

...................................................

...................................................

...................................................

...................................................

...................................................

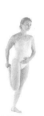

# Spine Stretch

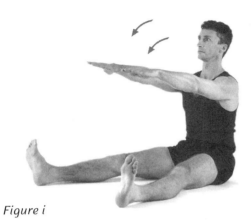

*Figure i*

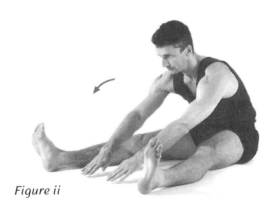

*Figure ii*

**PREREQUISITES:** The Start Stretches (Exercises 3 through 6a), stretches for hamstrings and thighs (Exercises 9-1 through 13).

**PURPOSE:** To stretch the spine and the hamstrings.

### EXERCISE DESCRIPTION:

*Starting Position:* Sit upright on the sitz bones with the legs slightly wider apart than shoulder distance, feet flexed, knees pressed to the floor. Lift the arms so that they are perpendicular to the ceiling (upper arms next to your ears), lifting the ribs vertically from the hips and drawing the shoulder blades toward the hips. Engage the B-Line Core.

a) Ocean breathe out to curl the chin down to the rib cage, then curl the nose toward the B-Line. Lower the arms, extending them in front of you as far forward as possible without hunching the shoulders, keeping the eyes to the floor (Figure i).

b) Breathe in to hold the position, pressing the hands into the floor.

c) Ocean breathe out to lengthen the spine forward as far as possible, chest toward ankles (Figure ii).

d) Breathe in to hold the stretch, pressing the hands into the floor.

e) Ocean breathe out to scoop the abdominals and curl the spine back to the upright position, imprinting onto an imaginary wall, still reaching through the fingertips as far forward as possible.

### KEY POINTS:

1. If you feel any discomfort in the back of the knees or cannot sit upright, bend the knees or sit on a folded towel.

2. Keep the shoulder blades pressed into the pocket.

3. Scoop the abdominals and imprint the spine on the return to the upright position. Start by engaging the B-Line Core, then stack the vertebrae one at a time on top of each other, lifting the ribs away from the hips, and keeping the chin lightly on the chest until the very end. Then lengthen through the crown of the head toward the ceiling.

# Spine Stretch *(cont'd.)*

4. Focus on breathing deeply into the armpits and upper back at all times.

5. Do not force the movement. As you complete more repetitions, you will gradually become looser.

6. *Simpler Version:* Start with the hands on the floor between the legs, elbows locked straight. Walk the fingers forward. Continue with the stretch as above. When returning upright, slide the hands on the floor back to the starting position.

**REPETITIONS:** One set of ten stretches.

**BREATHING REVIEW:** Ocean breathe out to curl the nose toward the B-Line and extend forward. Breathe in to hold the position.

Ocean breathe out to stretch forward.

Breathe in to hold. Ocean breathe out to return to the upright position.

*Notes*

.................................................

.................................................

.................................................

.................................................

.................................................

.................................................

.................................................

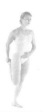

# Open Leg Rocker

**PREREQUISITES:** The Start Stretches (Exercises 3 through 6a), Hamstring Stretches (Exercises 9-1 through 10), The Perfect Abdominal Curl (Exercise 25), The Roll-Over (Exercise 34).

**PURPOSE:** To improve balance and control.

### EXERCISE DESCRIPTION:

*Starting Position:* Sit tall on the floor with your knees bent open, toes pointed and close to your tailbone, hands on the ankles and elbows resting lightly inside the open knees (Figure i).

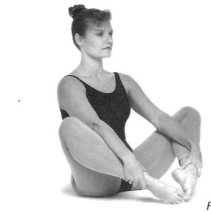

*Figure i*

a) Engage the B-Line Core and, balancing on your tailbone, straighten your legs into the air, one at a time, to form a V. Keep the arms as straight as possible (Figure ii).

b) Maintaining the V, curve your back into a C shape by sinking into your hips (with control), and breathe in to smoothly roll along your spine to the top of your shoulders (Figure iii).

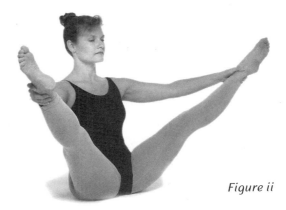

*Figure ii*

c) Sharp ocean breathe out (blast) to roll back to the upright position, sitting tall, chin up, spine long. Repeat the exercise from the starting position.

### KEY POINTS:

A great deal of balance and abdominal control are required for this exercise.

1. When the legs are extended into the air, try to align the toes with the top of your head.

2. Draw the hips toward the ribs on the roll-over and the ribs toward the hips on the roll-up.

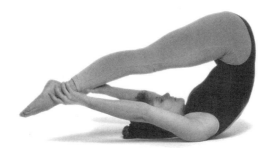

*Figure iii*

---

# Open Leg Rocker *(cont'd.)*

3. On the roll-up, flatten the ribs to reach the upright position, as if you had a rod through your spine from the tailbone to the crown of your head.

4. Roll over only onto the top of the shoulders, keeping your chin drawn softly to the chest.

5. If you feel unbalanced as you roll into the upright position, bend the knees slightly to gain more control over the movement.

6. Roll smoothly through the spine. If there are "flat spots" along the spine, bend the knees and take hold behind them.

**BEGINNER'S HINT:** If you are unable to gain control when doing this movement, try the following: From the starting position, try to straighten the legs open into the V position, one leg at a time; then ocean breathe out to bring the legs together, lowering the toes to touch the floor and trying to lift out of the lower back. Keeping your balance, breathe in to open the legs, sitting taller and lifting the ribs toward the toes. Ocean breathe out to bend the knees back to the starting position. Repeat six to ten times.

**REPETITIONS:** One set of six.

**BREATHING REVIEW:** Breathe in to extend the legs, ocean breathe out to sink into the hips, then breathe in to roll back. Ocean breathe out to roll upright.

*Notes*

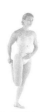

# Corkscrew: Basic

**PREREQUISITE:** The Hundreds: Alternating Legs (Exercise 31).

**PURPOSE:** To increase oblique and abdominal strength, as well as hip and lower-back mobility.

### EXERCISE DESCRIPTION:

*Starting Position:* Lie on your back on the floor and decompress the spine. Place your arms by your sides, palms down. Extend both legs vertically into the air, feet pointed and legs turned out, and squeeze the backs of the knees together.

a) Engage the B-Line Core, and ocean breathe out to lower both legs to the right side and then away from the body so that they are fully extended (but remaining raised off the ground), and then around to the left side. You're making a circle with your legs in one smooth, continuous motion.

b) Breathe in to return the legs to the vertical position.

c) Keep the B-Line Core engaged, and ocean breathe out to reverse the direction of the legs, lowering to the left this time. Again, breathe in to return the legs to the vertical position. Repeat the exercise, changing directions each time.

   Because of the continual change of direction, the obliques and abdominals are required to change their direction of control. This constant redirection of the muscle provides a greater challenge than doing ten circles in one direction.

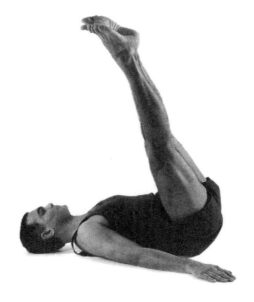

### KEY POINTS:

1. As the legs lower away from the body, flatten the rib cage to prevent the back from arching.

2. Imagine that the movement is being performed from the inner thighs near the groin: this will give you more control.

3. Keep the shoulders on the ground with the hands slightly away from the body.

4. Start with small corkscrews, without lifting the hips off the floor; then, as you gain more confidence and control, make the corkscrews bigger, still keeping the imaginary sacrum coin pressed to the floor.

**REPETITIONS:** One set of six to ten in each direction.

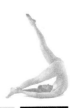

# Corkscrew 1: Intermediate

This exercise is similar in all aspects to the basic Corkscrew, except the circle is bigger.

**EXERCISE DESCRIPTION:** Make the circle bigger to work the abdominals more intensely. As this becomes easier, lift the arms out and away from the body, turning the palms up. If the palms are down, there is more tendency to push the hands against the floor to maintain control, rather than using the abdominals; this would also strain the neck and shoulders. As you become more proficient with this version, continue extending the arms until they are above shoulder height on the floor; keep the leg circle close to the floor. Keep the elbows and the shoulders on the floor at all times. This is abdominal control at its best.

*Notes*

........................................................

........................................................

........................................................

........................................................

........................................................

........................................................

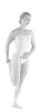

# Corkscrew 2: Advanced

**PREREQUISITES:** Corkscrew: Basic (Exercise 47-1), The Roll-Over (Exercise 34).

**PURPOSE:** To strengthen the abdominals, obliques, and spine, and to mobilize the spine and hips.

### EXERCISE DESCRIPTION:

*Starting Position:* Lie flat on your back on the floor and decompress the spine. Raise the legs to a vertical position, turned out and with feet pointed. Squeeze the backs of the knees together, and keep your arms by your sides, palms down (Figure i).

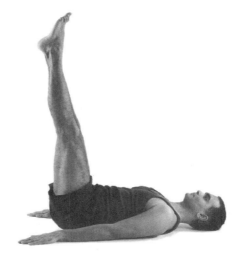

*Figure i*

a) Ocean breathe out to roll onto the shoulders in the roll-over position, as in Exercise 34 (Figure ii).

b) Hold the position for the breath in.

c) Ocean breathe out to take the legs to the right side of the body, rolling the hips to the left (Figure iii). Roll onto the right side of the body, and then onto your back, lowering the legs and making a circle with them in a smooth, continuous motion. Flatten the ribs to keep the back from arching excessively. There will be a slight arch in the back.

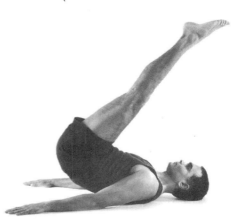

*Figure ii*

d) Breathe in to roll back up onto the left side of the body and again into the roll-over position.

e) Ocean breathe out to reverse the movement, rolling onto the left side of the body.

### KEY POINTS:

1. The farther into the roll-over you are at the beginning, the better. However, go no farther over than the top of the shoulders.

2. Squeeze the B-Line Core at all times.

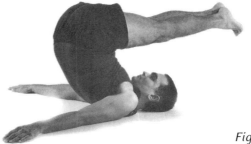

*Figure iii*

# Corkscrew 2: Advanced *(cont'd.)*

3. The bigger the circle (out to the sides and down to the floor), the more challenging the exercise.

4. Keep the movement fluid and the roll smooth.

5. Try to place the least amount of pressure possible on the hands. Keep the shoulders relaxed and down.

6. Keep the legs turned out, stretching through the toes as if drawing circles on the ceiling.

7. If the back arches too much, or the shoulders do most of the work, reduce the size of the circle.

8. Keep the back of the neck long and pressed into the mat.

9. Keep the shoulder blades drawn into the pocket.

**REPETITIONS:** Up to five complete movements (one complete corkscrew is a roll onto the side in each direction).

**BREATHING REVIEW:** Ocean breathe out to roll the back to the floor and stretch the legs away from the torso. Breathe in to roll onto the shoulders with the legs above the head.

**NOTE:** It may be a good idea to review the notes on breathing. See "General Breathing Rules" in Chapter 2.

*Notes*

......................................................

......................................................

......................................................

......................................................

......................................................

......................................................

......................................................

......................................................

......................................................

......................................................

......................................................

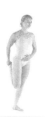

# The Saw

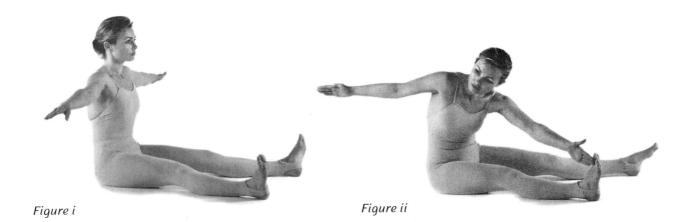

*Figure i*

*Figure ii*

**PREREQUISITE:** Spine Stretch (Exercise 45).

**PURPOSE:** To provide basic rotation of the spine, concentrating on the rib cage.

### EXERCISE DESCRIPTION:

*Starting Position:* Sit upright on the floor as if there were a rod through your spine. Extend the arms out to the sides, parallel to the floor, reaching through the fingertips, as if a pole were extended from one fingertip through the shoulders to the other fingertip. Squeeze the B-Line Core (Figure i).

a) Ocean breathe out to rotate the torso to the right by turning the rib cage and at the same time reaching forward with the left hand toward the outside of the right foot (Figure ii).

b) Keep breathing out to imitate a sawing action with the edge of the left hand halfway up the outside edge of the foot for two short strokes. Taking two sharper breaths out (percussion breaths) for each of the sawing movements will help you to stretch farther. Look toward the back (right) hand, which should be pointed to the corner of the ceiling behind you.

c) Breathe in to return to the upright position by rolling the rib cage back, using the oblique muscles and squeezing the Core.

d) Stretch to one side, then return to the upright position. Stretch to the other side with a continuous, flowing movement, then return again to the upright position.

### KEY POINTS:

1. As you reach forward to "saw off" the foot, rotate the torso as if you were trying to turn your chest toward the ceiling.

2. Lengthen through the crown of the head while reaching the chest along the thigh.

3. Press the opposite hip firmly into the floor at all times to keep the pelvis stable.

4. Keep the feet flexed.

5. If you cannot reach the foot, do not force the stretch. Reach instead to the outside of the calf. Some people may only be able to stretch about half as far as what is shown in the photograph. That's fine. Progress gradually from the point you find comfortable.

# The Saw *(cont'd.)*

6. For the two extra stretches with the percussion breaths, visualize going "far," then "farther."

**REPETITIONS:** Up to ten stretches on each side, alternating sides.

**BREATHING REVIEW:** Ocean breathe out to rotate and reach, and take an extra percussion breath out to reach far, then farther. Squeeze the Core and breathe in to rotate back to the upright position.

*Notes*

. . . . . . . . . . . . . . . . . . . . . . . . . . . . . . . . . . . . . . . . . . . . . . . . . . . . . . .

. . . . . . . . . . . . . . . . . . . . . . . . . . . . . . . . . . . . . . . . . . . . . . . . . . . . . . .

. . . . . . . . . . . . . . . . . . . . . . . . . . . . . . . . . . . . . . . . . . . . . . . . . . . . . . .

. . . . . . . . . . . . . . . . . . . . . . . . . . . . . . . . . . . . . . . . . . . . . . . . . . . . . . .

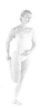

# Side Kick 1

**PREREQUISITES:** The Start Stretches (Exercises 3 through 6a), The Hundreds: Alternating Legs (Exercise 31).

**PURPOSE:** To mobilize the hips, stretch the hamstrings, and strengthen the lower back.

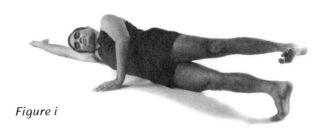

*Figure i*

### EXERCISE DESCRIPTION:

*Starting Position:* Lie on the floor on your right side, balancing on your right hip, with your head resting on your extended right arm, right elbow in line with the body, and left hand palm down on the mat by your waist. Engage the B-Line Core.

a) Keeping your legs straight, bring them slightly forward, with both feet flexed and lengthened through the heels. Turn the right leg out and press the right toes into the floor. Lift the left leg slightly to hip level, keep the foot flexed, and squeeze the B-Line Core (Figure i).

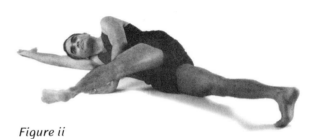

*Figure ii*

b) Take a deep breath in to kick the left leg forward as far as you can, pressing through the heel. Keep the spine straight (Figure ii).

c) At the end of the kick, do a further, smaller kick, inhaling an extra breath to expand the lungs more.

d) Point your foot and ocean breathe out to kick your leg back in a sweeping motion, stretching through the top of the thigh and keeping the B-Line Core engaged (Figure iii). Flatten the rib cage and keep the back as straight as you can.

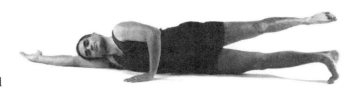

*Figure iii*

e) Flex the foot and press through the heel for the next kick forward.

Repeat on the other side.

# Side Kick 1 *(cont'd.)*

### KEY POINTS:

1. Stabilize your center by squeezing the Core.

2. As if your hip were the center of a circle, lengthen through the heel and then the toes, reaching past the outer rim of the circle.

3. Keep the shoulders stable, with the top shoulder blade drawn into the pocket. Keep the chin lifted.

4. Lengthen through the crown of the head.

5. To keep the top hip directly above the bottom one, create a small gap between the waist and the floor.

6. If you feel any strain in the back, do not sweep the leg back as far.

7. If you feel the hipbone on the mat, place a flat cushion under the hip.

**REPETITIONS:** Ten kicks on each side.

**BREATHING REVIEW:** Breathe in to kick forward, and take an extra breath in at the stretch. Ocean breathe out to sweep the leg back.

*Notes*

.................................................

.................................................

.................................................

.................................................

.................................................

.................................................

.................................................

.................................................

.................................................

.................................................

.................................................

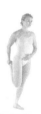

# Side Leg Lifts

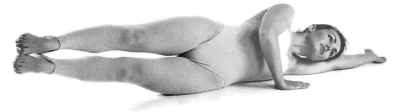

**PREREQUISITE:** The Hundreds: Alternating Legs (Exercise 31).

**PURPOSE:** To strengthen the side muscles of the waist (quadratus lumborum), the obliques, the muscles of the outside of the thigh (tensor fascia lata), and the adductors.

### EXERCISE DESCRIPTION:

*Starting Position:* Lie on your left side with your head resting on your extended left arm, palm to the ceiling, elbow in line with the body. Place the right hand or fingertips lightly on the floor next to the waist. Keep the legs parallel, slightly in front of the body, with the toes pointed. There should be a small gap between the left side of the waist and the floor. Tuck the pelvis to assist in supporting the lower back.

a) Engage the B-Line Core and ocean breathe out to lift both legs as high as you can without leaning the hips backward, squeezing the inner thigh of the bottom leg.

b) Breathe in to lower the legs slowly until they almost touch the floor (90 percent). Repeat the exercise.

### KEY POINTS:

1. Maintain the gap between the waistband and the floor.

2. Start the ocean breath out just before beginning the movement.

3. For beginners, to prevent the hips from rolling back, keep your back flat against a wall without leaning against it.

4. If there is an arch in the back, flatten it by engaging the lower abdominals more with a pelvic tuck.

5. Keep the supporting hand relaxed—do not use it to push on the floor, as this will hunch the shoulder.

6. For more control and toning of the adductor muscles, place a thin cushion between the thighs and squeeze as you lift.

7. If you feel pressure on the bottom hip as you lift the legs, place a flat cushion under the hip.

**REPETITIONS:** Ten lifts, then change and repeat on the other side.

**INCREASE THE CHALLENGE:** Place your free hand (the one you're not lying on) behind your head, with the elbow pointed toward the ceiling. Greater balance is required for this version.

### VARIATION—SIDE LEG KICK UP:

Lie in the same starting position as for the Side Leg Lifts (Exercise 50).

a) Turn out the top leg so the kneecap is facing the ceiling, and point the foot.

b) Engage the B-Line Core and breathe in to kick the top leg up toward the ceiling. Do not lean back.

c) Flex the top foot and ocean breathe out to press through the heel, lowering the top foot 90 percent of the way back toward the other foot. Repeat ten times, then change sides.

# Pelvic Curl

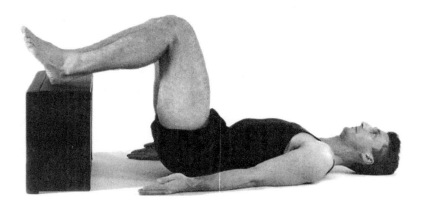

**PREREQUISITE:** None.

**PURPOSE:** To help open and mobilize the lower back, and to connect the lower abdominals.

**EXERCISE DESCRIPTION:** This exercise is best done with the legs on a chair.

*Starting Position:* Lie on your back with your feet on a chair, hip distance apart. Decompress the spine. The thigh bone should be at a ninety-degree angle to the floor.

a) With your arms lying palm up by your sides, engage the B-Line Core and ocean breathe out to draw the hipbones toward the rib cage, peeling the lower back off the floor. Continue to do so until the pelvis tilts off the floor about two to four inches.

b) Breathe in to slowly release the hips back down to the floor, imprinting the spine. Maintain the B-Line Core throughout the movement.

**KEY POINTS:**

1. It may help to gently press the fingers of one hand into the lower abdominals to feel the connection of the abdominal muscles.

2. Do not press downward with the arms or feet to achieve the movement.

3. Lengthen through the crown of the head.

4. To relax the shoulders, slide the hands past the hips when both curling up and imprinting down.

**REPETITIONS:** Two sets of ten repetitions.

*Notes*

..............................................................

..............................................................

..............................................................

..............................................................

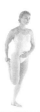

# Pelvic Lift

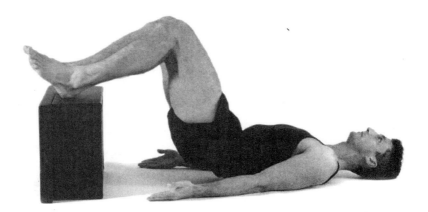

**PREREQUISITE AND PURPOSE:** Same as for the Pelvic Curl (Exercise 51). This exercise will also strengthen and tighten the buttocks.

**EXERCISE DESCRIPTION:** The Pelvic Lift starts in the same position as the Pelvic Curl. Its movements are the same as well, except you lift the pelvis higher.

a) After you have achieved the Pelvic Curl, continue breathing out to peel the spine off the floor until the spine is raised all the way up to the shoulders. Do not arch the lower back; you should feel no pressure in the spine. Control all the work from the B-Line Core.

b) When releasing the position, breathe in to imprint the spine onto the floor one vertebra at a time.

**KEY POINTS:**

Same as for the Pelvic Curl. In addition:

1. The knees should be hip distance apart and at a right angle above the navel when in the resting position.

2. Remember to peel the spine off the floor and to imprint it back on the floor.

3. Do not peel the spine off any higher than is comfortable, and do not allow the back to arch.

**REPETITIONS:** One set of ten repetitions.

*Notes*

.............................................

.............................................

.............................................

.............................................

# Teaser 1: Basic

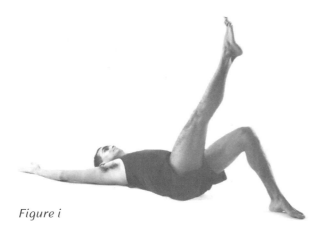

*Figure i*

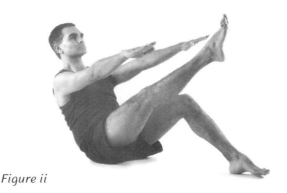

*Figure ii*

**PREREQUISITES:** The Hundreds: Alternating Legs (Exercise 31), The Perfect Abdominal Curl (Exercise 25), The Roll-Over (Exercise 34).

**PURPOSE:** To strengthen the abdominals through a continuous movement.

### EXERCISE DESCRIPTION:

*Starting Position:* Lie on your back with your knees bent and feet flat on the floor. Decompress the spine. Extend the arms on the floor above the head. Extend one leg into the air, keeping both knees at approximately the same level (Figure i).

a) Breathe in to draw your hands toward your thighs, keeping them shoulder distance apart, till they are positioned just above the B-Line. Lift the head off the floor.

b) Start the ocean breath out to roll your spine off the mat in a long curve like the arch of a bow, keeping the neck long.

c) As you come up to the highest point, without putting any pressure on the feet, extend the fingers farther toward a line above the toes of the leg that's extended. Avoid rounding the shoulders.

d) Breathe in to straighten your back, opening the chest; lift the ribs toward the knees, and sit tall on the sitz bones (Figure ii).

e) Ocean breathe out to imprint your spine back onto the mat, starting with a very small posterior pelvic tuck (or sinking into the hips), looking into the groin. Keep the back curved like the curve of a long bow, and move back to the starting position.

f) Do not rest. Keep all the muscles engaged and move immediately to the next repetition.

### KEY POINTS:

1. Flatten the ribs before the lift, to keep the ribs and upper abdominals in a flat line throughout the movement.

2. Keep the shoulder blades pressed into the pocket, and lengthen through the crown of the head.

3. Lift tall out of the hips as if you were trying to extend the lower back. Lift the ribs toward the knee.

4. If you feel the tops of the thighs overworking, do fewer repetitions or do some Thigh Stretches (Exercises 11 through 13) before continuing.

**REPETITIONS:** Up to eight repetitions on each side.

**BREATHING REVIEW:** Ocean breathe out to lift the torso, and breathe in to grow taller. Breathe out to lower back to the floor.

**INCREASE THE CHALLENGE:** Lie on your back with both feet resting lightly on a box or high chair, legs straight and parallel and extended at approximately a forty-five-degree angle to the floor, feet softly pointed. Keep your arms above your head on the floor. Continue as in steps a through f above.

*Notes*

....................................................

....................................................

....................................................

....................................................

....................................................

....................................................

# Teaser 2

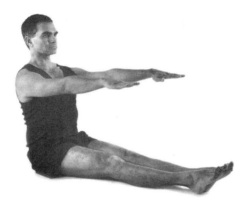 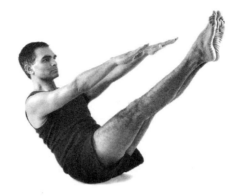

**PREREQUISITE:** Teaser 1: Basic (Exercise 53-1).

**PURPOSE:** To increase abdominal strength, hip mobility, and hip flexor control, and to stretch the lower back.

### EXERCISE DESCRIPTION:

*Starting Position:* Sit tall on your sitz bones, legs extended parallel on the ground, toes pointed. Your arms should be extended forward at shoulder level, palms down.

a) Engage the B-Line Core and breathe in to lean the torso back at a forty-five-degree angle as you raise the legs into a V sit-up. Lift the feet until they are level with your head (or as close as you can), balancing on your sitz bones. See if you can touch your toes to your fingers, keeping the back straight, the shoulder blades drawn into the pocket, and the neck long.

b) Pause for a second, consolidating the strength of the abdominals and the firm lengthening of the torso. Squeeze the inner thighs together.

c) Ocean breathe out to lower the legs to just off the floor, extending through the toes.

d) Breathe in to return to the starting position. Do not rest.

e) Repeat.

### KEY POINTS:

1. Keep the shoulder blades drawn into the pocket and the neck in line with the upper back.

2. Keep the ribs flat when lowering the legs.

3. Stretch through the crown of the head, through the fingertips, and through the point of the toes.

**REPETITIONS:** Same as for Exercise 53-1.

*Notes*

. . . . . . . . . . . . . . . . . . . . . . . . . . . . . . . . . . . . . . . . . . . . . . . . . . .

. . . . . . . . . . . . . . . . . . . . . . . . . . . . . . . . . . . . . . . . . . . . . . . . . . .

. . . . . . . . . . . . . . . . . . . . . . . . . . . . . . . . . . . . . . . . . . . . . . . . . . .

. . . . . . . . . . . . . . . . . . . . . . . . . . . . . . . . . . . . . . . . . . . . . . . . . . .

# Teaser 3

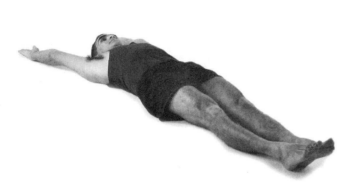
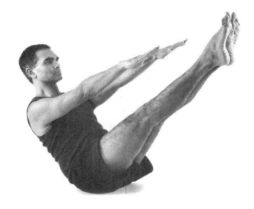

**PREREQUISITE:** Teaser 2 (Exercise 53-2).

**PURPOSE:** To increase balance and control.

### EXERCISE DESCRIPTION:

*Starting Position:* Lie on your back (supine), legs extended on the ground and parallel, with feet pointed. Extend the arms through the fingertips above the head, shoulder width apart.

a) Engage the B-Line Core and ocean breathe out to lift the legs, arms, and torso in one movement into a V sit-up position.

b) Breathe in to balance on your sitz bones, reaching for the toes with the fingers. Keep the back as upright as possible, as if there were a rod in your spine. Keep the neck long.

c) Breathe out to slightly tuck the pelvis, contracting the abdominals. Slowly elongate the torso, legs, and arms back onto the mat at the same time, to the starting position.

**INCREASE THE CHALLENGE:** When you have lifted the legs, extend the arms overhead toward the ceiling, in line with your ears, drawing the shoulder blades into the pocket. Then continue with step c above, keeping the hands extended toward the ceiling.

**KEY POINTS:** Same as for Teaser 1: Basic (Exercise 53-1).

**REPETITIONS:** Up to ten repetitions.

### Notes

..........................................................

..........................................................

..........................................................

..........................................................

..........................................................

..........................................................

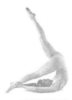

# Leg Pull Prone

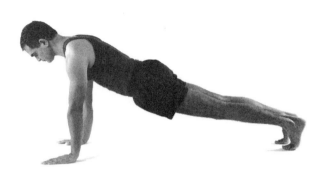 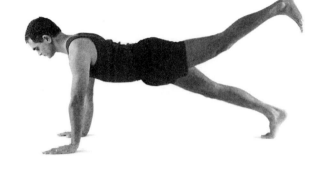

**PREREQUISITE:** The Hundreds: Alternating Legs (Exercise 31).

**PURPOSE:** To open the hip joints and strengthen the lower back and shoulders.

### EXERCISE DESCRIPTION:

*Starting Position:* Assume a push-up position: arms locked, fingers pointing forward, and shoulders, hips, and heels in a straight line.

a) Engage the B-Line Core with a slight pelvic tuck to help connect the lower abdominals and the buttocks. Keep the neck long and in a straight line with the back. Press the heels toward the floor as far as you can. Tighten the buttocks.

b) Breathe in to lift the left leg as high as you can toward the ceiling with the foot flexed hard and the knee joint locked, without allowing the hips to move or the back to arch.

c) Ocean breathe out to softly lower the leg to the floor, lengthening farther through the heel. Change legs.

**INCREASE THE CHALLENGE:** At the top of the leg lift, do a double kick upward with an extra breath out.

### KEY POINTS:

1. Breathe in to extend the leg upward, squeezing the Core and tucking the pelvis.

2. Consciously feel the abdominals tighten and support the entire body. Lengthen simultaneously through the crown of the head and through the heels. Stay in a straight line from head to heels.

3. Keep your weight balanced between the big toe and the second toe.

4. Keep the elbows lengthened and locked or slightly bent, but do not hyperextend them, as doing so may cause a strain at the elbow joint.

**REPETITIONS:** One set of five repetitions on each leg.

**BREATHING REVIEW:** Breathe in to lift the leg. Ocean breathe out to lower the leg.

# Leg Pull Supine

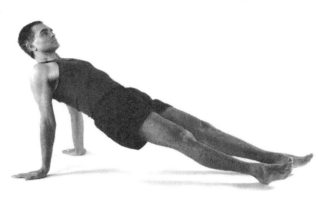 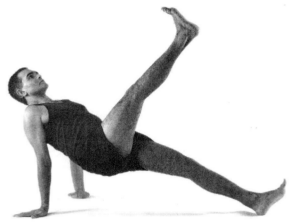

**PREREQUISITES:** Hamstring Stretch 2 (Exercise 9-2), Thigh Stretch 3: Kneeling (Exercise 13), Leg Pull Prone (Exercise 54).

**PURPOSE:** To mobilize the hip joints, stretch the hamstrings, and stabilize the shoulders.

### EXERCISE DESCRIPTION:

*Starting Position:* Sit on the mat with your hands behind you, fingers facing backwards, legs extended in front. Lift the hips off the ground. Keep the shoulders, hips, and heels in a straight line, the toes pointed, the eyes to the ceiling, the pelvis slightly tucked under (posteriorly), and the shoulder blades pressed into the pocket.

a) Engage the B-Line Core and flex your right foot. Breathe in to kick the right leg toward the ceiling (past the vertical line if you can), squeezing the Core tighter. Keep the hips pressed toward the ceiling, lift the chest toward the ceiling, and lengthen the back of the neck. Keep the shoulders relaxed, the ribs drawn toward the hips, and the abdominals firm.

b) Point the foot of the raised leg and ocean breathe out to slowly lower the leg to the floor.

c) Touch the foot lightly on the floor and kick the same leg again.

**INCREASE THE CHALLENGE:** At the top of the kick, do a double kick and take a double breath in.

### KEY POINTS:

1. Keep the pelvis lifted as the leg kicks up.

2. Elongate the head and neck out of the shoulders.

3. Be sure that the pressure on the supporting leg is in the center of the heel.

4. Imagine there is a rod extending from the top and center point of your shoulders to the tailbone, and another across your shoulders.

5. Avoid hyperextending the elbows.

**REPETITIONS:** Five kicks with one leg, then five kicks with the other.

**BREATHING REVIEW:** Breathe in on the kick up, and ocean breathe out on the return.

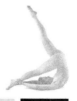

# Side Kick 2

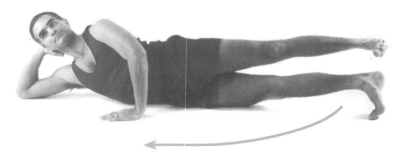

**PREREQUISITES:** The Start Stretches (Exercises 3 through 6a), The Hundreds: Alternating Legs (Exercise 31), Side Kick 1 (Exercise 49).

**PURPOSE:** To mobilize the hips, stretch the thighs, and strengthen the lower back.

### EXERCISE DESCRIPTION:

*Starting Position:* Lie on the floor on your right side, and rest your head on your right hand.

a) Keeping your legs straight and parallel, bring them slightly forward, with both feet flexed and the bottom leg turned out and the toes pressed into the floor. Lengthen through the heels. Lift the top leg slightly, to hip level, keeping the foot flexed, and engage the B-Line Core.

b) Take a deep ocean breath out to kick the top leg forward as far as you can, pressing through the heel. Keep the spine straight. At the end of the kick, do an additional, smaller kick, exhaling an extra breath to kick farther.

c) Point your foot and breathe in to kick the top leg back in a sweeping motion. As the leg sweeps behind the straight line of the body, raise the torso, placing your weight on the right elbow and creating a large gap under your right armpit.

d) Flex the foot and press through the heel for the next kick forward. As the leg kicks forward again, lean back slightly to reduce the gap under the armpit, keeping the back as straight as possible, and flatten the rib cage.

**INCREASE THE CHALLENGE:** For the starting position, place your left hand behind your head, with the elbow pointing toward the ceiling and in line with the body.

### KEY POINTS:

1. Stabilize your center by squeezing the Core.

2. Imagine that your hip is the center of a circle, and lengthen through the heel and then the toe, reaching past the outer rim of the circle.

3. Keep the shoulders stable and the chin lifted. Lengthen through the crown of the head. To keep the top hip directly above the bottom one, create a small gap between the waist and the floor.

4. If you feel any strain in the back, do not sweep the leg back as far.

5. Do not allow the ribs to protrude forward.

6. If you feel the hipbone on the mat, place a flat cushion under the hip.

**REPETITIONS:** Ten kicks on each side.

**BREATHING REVIEW:** Breathe out to kick forward, taking an extra breath out for an extra stretch. Breathe in to sweep the leg back.

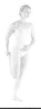

# Boomerang

**PREREQUISITES:** Teaser 2 (Exercise 53-2), The Roll-Over (Exercise 34).

**PURPOSE:** To gain control and mobilization of the spine, shoulders, and hips, and to stretch the hamstrings.

### EXERCISE DESCRIPTION:

*Starting Position:* Sit upright on the floor and engage the B-Line Core, imagining that you have a rod through your spine. Place your palms on the floor by your hips, fingers forward, and extend your legs forward, with the right leg and ankle crossed over the left.

a) Tuck the pelvis slightly, take a deep breath out to sink into your hips, and roll over, drawing the thighs toward the ribs until the feet almost touch the mat. Lengthen the neck and roll only to the top of the shoulders (Figure i).

b) Breathe out to roll the spine back onto the floor, lifting the torso at the same time. Lift your hands off the floor and behind your back, holding the left hand with the right, keeping the elbows straight. Continue to extend the hands behind you away from your back.

c) Breathe in to balance on your sitz bones for three seconds with the legs high off the floor, spine erect, legs straight (Figure ii).

d) Ocean breathe out to continue the roll forward, lengthening your chest toward your knees and your head toward your feet, with your hands extended behind you and pressing toward the ceiling (Figure iii).

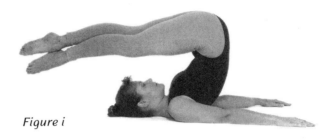

*Figure i*

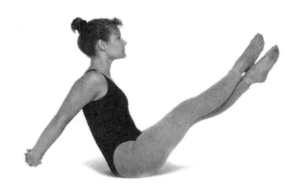

*Figure ii*

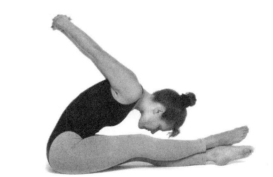

*Figure iii*

# Boomerang *(cont'd.)*

e) Breathe in to release the hands and stretch them around in a circle to the front of the body and then toward the ceiling, rotating the shoulder joints. Reach forward and hold onto the feet (or ankles or shins, if you can't reach the feet) for a stretch.

f) Breathe out to scoop and curl the torso into the upright sitting position, placing the hands on the floor by the hips, and cross the legs over the other way (left over right).

### KEY POINTS:

1. The entire movement centers around contracted and controlled abdominal strength, precision, and flowing movement.

2. Roll over only onto the tops of the shoulders.

3. Keep the shoulder blades pressed into the pocket.

4. Lift the ribs away from the hips and keep the neck straight and long when clasping the hands behind the back.

**REPETITIONS:** One set of up to eight complete movements.

**BREATHING REVIEW:** Breathe in to sit tall, and ocean breathe out to roll over. Breathe in to uncross and recross the legs the other way. Breathe out to roll up to balance. Breathe in to hold for three seconds. Ocean breathe out to roll forward and reach the chest to the knees. Breathe in to circle the arms forward. Breathe out to curl to the upright position.

*Notes*

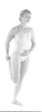

# Seal

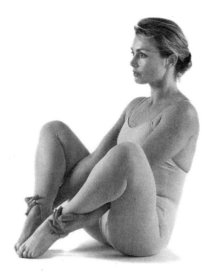

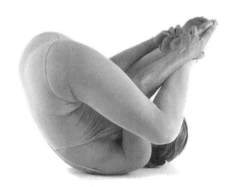

**PREREQUISITE:** The Roll-Over (Exercise 34).

**PURPOSE:** To gain balance and control of movement, and to stretch the spine.

### EXERCISE DESCRIPTION:

*Starting Position:* Sit tall on the mat, with the knees bent and open, the elbows placed on the insides of the thighs, the forearms under the calves, and the hands holding onto the fronts of the ankles. Place the soles of the feet together and raise the heels off the mat. Keep the toes lightly touching the mat.

a) Engage the B-Line Core and ocean breathe out to tuck the pelvis and start to roll the spine.

b) Breathe in to continue smoothly rolling over onto the tops of the shoulders, until the feet are pointing toward the wall above the head—not on the floor.

c) Balancing in this position, open the feet eight inches and clap the soles of the feet together twice.

d) Ocean breathe out to roll into the starting position, straightening the spine at the top of the roll, toes just off the mat, and clap the soles of the feet three times.

### KEY POINTS:

1. Keep the neck long, and keep the ribs drawn toward the hips on the roll back.

2. When balancing on the shoulders, keep the abdominals hollow and firm, squeezing the Core.

3. Keep the shoulder blades pressed into the pocket to avoid neck strain.

4. Stay off the neck by lifting the feet toward the ceiling.

**REPETITIONS:** One set of up to eight repetitions.

**BREATHING REVIEW:** Breathe out to sit in a continuous C curve. Breathe in to roll back onto the shoulders. Loudly ocean breathe out to roll up.

# Control Balance

**PREREQUISITE:** The Roll-Over (Exercise 34).

**PURPOSE:** To gain control, balance, coordination, and abdominal strength.

### EXERCISE DESCRIPTION:

*Starting Position:* Lie on your back with your arms above your head on the floor. Decompress the spine. Lift the legs to a vertical position, keeping them straight and parallel.

a) Engage the B-Line Core and ocean breathe out to roll over until the toes are just off the mat, with the tailbone pointed to the ceiling. Hold on to the right ankle with both hands.

b) Breathe in to extend the left leg toward the ceiling, past the vertical line of the hip, extending through the toes. Keep the leg turned out and the foot pointed. Extend the spine as upright as possible, pressing the tailbone toward the ceiling.

c) Breathe out to release the right ankle, and smoothly scissor the legs, keeping the torso and legs under control. Keep the tailbone lengthened toward the ceiling.

d) Breathe in to extend the right leg, turned out and pointed, toward the ceiling. Holding onto the left ankle, and with the left leg straight, press the toes toward the spot on the ceiling that is directly above the crown of your head.

### KEY POINTS:

1. Keep the other leg extended toward the ceiling, straightening the knee joint.

2. Consciously think of releasing the front of the thigh.

3. Keep the shoulders open and on the mat, and the neck long.

4. Keep the abdominals hollow and the back straight.

**REPETITIONS:** One set of six extensions on each leg.

**BREATHING REVIEW:** Breathe in to extend the leg to the ceiling. Ocean breathe out to change the legs.

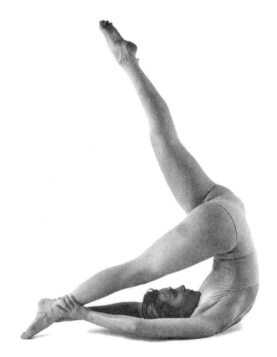

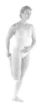

# 9

## THE ADVANCED ROUTINE

As small
bricks are
employed to
build large
buildings, so
will the
development
of small muscles
help develop
large muscles.

— J. PILATES

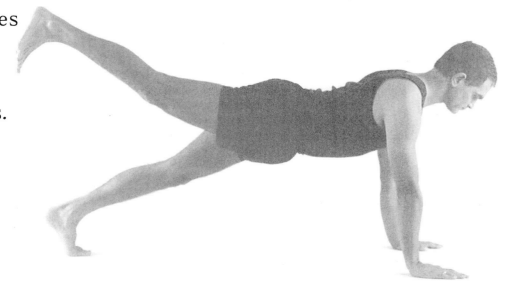

# The Hundreds: Lower and Raise

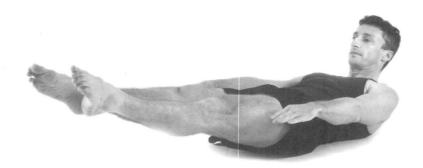

**PREREQUISITE:** The Hundreds: Alternating Legs (Exercise 31).

**PURPOSE:** To strengthen the abdominals with increased body extension.

**EXERCISE DESCRIPTION:** Start in the same position as for the Hundreds: Alternating Legs (Exercise 31). Keep the feet flexed and turned out.

a) Engage the B-Line Core, scoop the abdominals, and ocean breathe out to lower the legs toward the floor as low as possible for a count of five, keeping the imaginary lumbar coin pressed to the floor. At the same time, try to lift your buttocks off the floor for stronger lower-abdominal connection.

b) Point the feet, engage the B-Line Core more firmly, and breathe in to raise the legs back to the vertical position, squeezing the inner thighs together and pressing the sacrum into the floor.

**KEY POINTS:**

Same as those for the earlier Hundreds exercises (Exercise 31), as well as the following:

1. When lowering the legs, squeeze the inner thighs together and allow the abdominal muscles to slowly release; this will allow the legs to descend without arching the back.

2. Anchor the abdominals before lifting the legs, and imagine the hips drawing toward the ribs. The contraction of the abdominals is what brings the legs back to the vertical position.

3. Squeeze the inner thighs together. As you lower the legs, be sure to avoid lowering the head and shoulders, as doing so will arch the back (it might help to look in a mirror to check the stability of the torso).

4. Keep the abdominals scooped at all times.

5. Only do as many repetitions as are comfortable.

**REPETITIONS:** Two sets of ten, with a five-second rest between each set.

# Roll-Over: Bent Legs

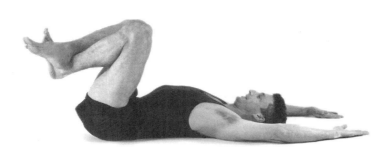

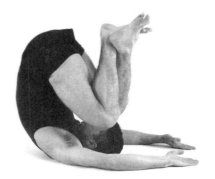

**PREREQUISITES:** The Roll-Over (Exercise 34), Rolling Like a Ball (Exercise 37).

**PURPOSE:** To connect the deeper abdominal muscles, especially in the lower-abdominal section.

### EXERCISE DESCRIPTION:

*Starting Position:* Lie on the floor with your back flat, and decompress the spine. Bend the knees to the chest, keeping them shoulder distance apart, and cross the ankles.

   a) Engage the B-Line, and while attempting to keep your heels as close as you can to your buttocks, ocean breathe out to roll the hips off the floor toward your ribs. Draw your knees close to your chest and in toward your armpits.

   b) Roll onto the shoulders only, lengthening the neck.

   c) Breathe into your upper back to hold the position.

   d) Ocean breathe out to slowly roll back down, imprinting your spine onto the floor, and slowly release the abdominals to prevent the head and shoulders from lifting off the floor.

### KEY POINTS:

1. If you are unable to perform the exercise with the heels to the tailbone, lengthen the legs until you gain more control. Start the exercise with your legs slightly extended and bent, ankles crossed. As you become more proficient, keep the heels closer to the tailbone.

2. It is on the roll down that you will feel the lower abdominals connecting.

3. Continue the repetitions without any rest. Keep the thighs close to the torso at all times.

4. Roll onto the shoulders only, not the neck.

**REPETITIONS:** One set of ten. After each roll, alternate the ankle that is on top.

### Notes

..........................................................

..........................................................

..........................................................

# Pendulum

**PREREQUISITE:** Corkscrew 2: Advanced (Exercise 47-3).

**PURPOSE:** To strengthen the obliques and the abdominals, and to mobilize and strengthen the spine.

### EXERCISE DESCRIPTION:

*Starting Position:* Lie on your back on the floor and decompress the spine. Extend the legs toward the ceiling, turned out and with feet pointed. Extend the arms above the head, elbows bent and pressed into the mat, and hands slightly more than shoulder distance apart. (In the basic version, the hands are by the sides, as shown in the figure.)

a) Engage the B-Line Core and, keeping the feet together, ocean breathe out to lower your legs to the right, keeping your toes in line with your navel and lifting the left hip off the floor. Keep the shoulder blades and elbows pressed into the mat. Turn the head toward the left.

b) Breathe in to draw the hips toward the ribs, and imprint the left side of the rib cage back onto the floor. Then continue with the rest of the spine until the left hip once again presses into the floor.

c) Keep moving the legs to the other side without stopping. Continue turning the head in the opposite direction from the legs.

### KEY POINTS:

1. Lower the legs as far as possible while still keeping the opposite shoulder on the mat. Release the chest muscle opposite from the side toward which the legs are lowering to allow the shoulder to stay on the mat.

2. Keep the legs turned out, especially when returning to the vertical position.

3. If there is too much pressure on the arms to raise the legs back to the vertical position, then the legs have gone over too far.

4. While the legs are still lowered, draw the legs slightly up toward the elbow to keep the abdominals engaged and prevent the back from arching. Keep the toes in line with the navel. As you develop more control, lower the legs farther, to a distance of several inches off the floor, without lifting the shoulder blades at all. Well done if you are able to accomplish this without straining!

**REPETITIONS:** One set of ten on each side, alternating sides.

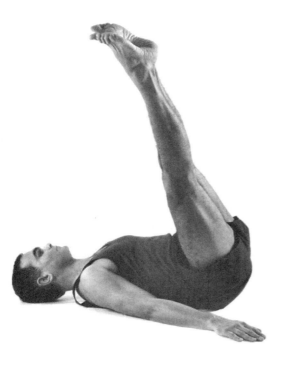

# Neck Curl

**PREREQUISITES:** The Hundreds: Lower and Raise (Exercise 60), The Perfect Abdominal Curl (Exercise 25) with straight legs.

**PURPOSE:** To improve abdominal control and strength.

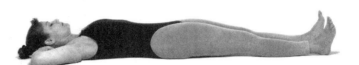

*Figure i*

### EXERCISE DESCRIPTION:

*Starting Position:* Lie on your back on the floor, legs together and extended in front of you, feet flexed, backs of the knees pressed into the floor. Place your hands behind your head, with the fingers and thumbs interlocked and your elbows on the mat (Figure i).

a) Engage the B-Line Core and breathe in to raise the head and shoulders off the mat, keeping the elbows behind the ears, as if a bar were passing in front of the elbows and behind the head (Figure ii).

b) Ocean breathe out to curl forward, contracting the ribs toward the hips, "zipping up" the stomach. Press your spine into the floor to come up. Reach forward as far as you can, trying to extend your chest to your knees.

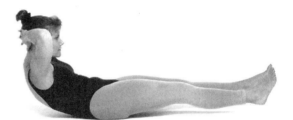

*Figure ii*

c) Breathe in to imprint your spine up an imaginary wall into the upright position. Lift the ribs out of the hips without hunching the shoulders (Figure iii). Keep shoulder blades drawn into the pocket.

d) Ocean breathe out to sink into the hips, tucking the pelvis to connect the lower abdominals, pressing through the heels, and imprinting your spine on the mat, curling the hips toward the ribs until the shoulder blades rest on the mat (Figure ii).

e) Extend the neck onto the mat, maintaining the B-Line Core.

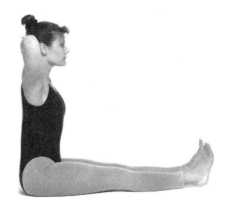

*Figure iii*

# Neck Curl *(cont'd.)*

## KEY POINTS:

1. Zip up the stomach before you start to lift the head.

2. Keep the elbows wide open.

3. Keep the shoulder blades pressed into the pocket.

4. Press the spine into the mat to come up.

5. Ocean breathe out 75 percent of your capacity during the first 25 percent of the movement up or down.

6. Flatten the ribs to the floor before rolling the shoulders off the mat.

7. Keep the chin slightly off the chest.

8. Do not pull on the neck.

**REPETITIONS:** One set of up to ten.

**BREATHING REVIEW:** Breathe in to lift the head and shoulders. Ocean breathe out to roll the torso up and forward. Breathe in to straighten up to the vertical position. Ocean breathe out to imprint the spine back onto the floor.

*Notes*

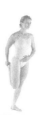

# Helicopter Hundreds

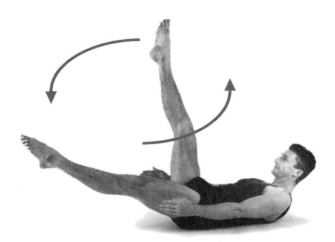

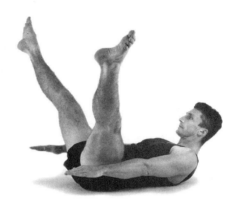

**PREREQUISITE:** The Hundreds: Alternating Legs (Exercise 31).

**PURPOSE:** To strengthen the abdominals and obliques. To mobilize the hip joints.

### EXERCISE DESCRIPTION:

*Starting Position:* Lie on your back on the floor and decompress the spine. Draw the knees to the chest and place the hands on the knees.

a) Engage the B-Line Core and ocean breathe out to contract forward, arms extended just off the floor to mid-thigh, elbows slightly bent. Gradually extend the legs vertically above the hips, with the feet pointed and legs turned out, eyes on the knees. Hold the position for a breath in.

b) Take two sharp breaths out to rapidly scissor (or split) the legs twice, keeping the left leg extended toward the ceiling and lowering the right leg to the floor, keeping the hips stable.

c) Breathe in to take the legs around in a circle in opposite directions, away from the body, keeping the legs turned out and the

feet pointed. The right leg opens to the side and comes up to the vertical position; the left leg opens to the side and lowers to just off the floor.

d) Repeat from step b above.

e) Repeat five times in each direction.

### KEY POINTS:

1. Lengthen out of the hip sockets as much as possible, maintaining your turnout.

2. Focus on the inner thigh (adductor) muscles to make the circle.

3. If the hip joints "click," either lengthen out of the hip joints further, reduce the range of movement when making the circle, or reduce the turnout of the leg.

**REPETITIONS:** Repeat five times, then change direction.

**BREATHING REVIEW:** Two rapid ocean breaths out to lower and "split" the legs twice. Breathe in to circle the legs.

# Jackknife

**PREREQUISITES:** Roll-Over: Bent Legs (Exercise 61), Helicopter Hundreds (Exercise 64), The Perfect Abdominal Curl (Exercise 25) with straight legs.

**PURPOSE:** To stretch the spine, stretch the neck, and increase abdominal control.

### EXERCISE DESCRIPTION:

*Starting Position:* Lie on your back, arms at your sides with palms down, and decompress the spine. Extend the legs vertically, toes pointed and parallel (Figure i).

a) Ocean breathe out to roll over onto the shoulders, taking the legs to a forty-five-degree angle from the floor (Figure ii).

b) Continue breathing out to immediately lengthen the legs to a vertical position, as if the body were in a straight line to the ceiling. Extend through the toes, squeeze the inner thighs together, and contract the buttocks firmly. Press your hips toward an imaginary line extending upward from your eyes (Figure iii).

c) Breathe in to stretch the feet higher to the ceiling.

d) Ocean breathe out to slowly imprint your spine on the mat, keeping your feet above your eyes until the hips have lengthened away from the ribs and pressed into the mat (Figure iv).

e) Breathe in to return the legs to vertical (starting position), pressing the imaginary sacrum coin into the floor.

f) Ocean breathe out to lower the legs toward the floor, but only as far as you can while still keeping the lumbar coin pressed into the floor.

g) Breathe in to raise the legs once again to vertical, hips down and inner thighs squeezed.

h) Repeat.

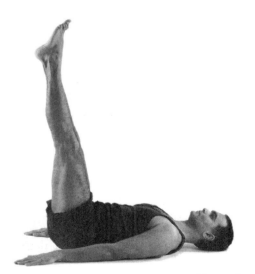

*Figure i*

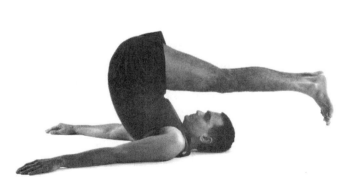

*Figure ii*

## KEY POINTS:

1. Keep the shoulders relaxed, without putting much pressure into the hands.

2. The initial part of the jackknife over and up is a fast movement, but you should come down from it slowly.

3. Squeeze the B-Line Core at all times to maintain strong abdominals.

4. Keep the neck as long as possible, by lengthening through the crown of the head.

**REPETITIONS:** One set of up to eight repetitions.

**BREATHING REVIEW:** Ocean breathe out to jack-knife over and up to the vertical position. Balance and breathe into the upper back to grow taller. Ocean breathe out to roll down.

*Notes*

...............................................

...............................................

...............................................

...............................................

...............................................

...............................................

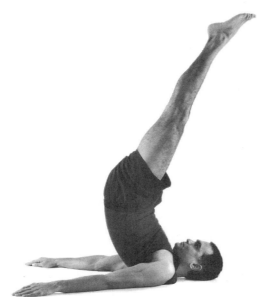

*Figure iii*

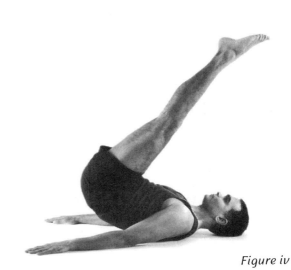

*Figure iv*

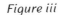

# Scissors

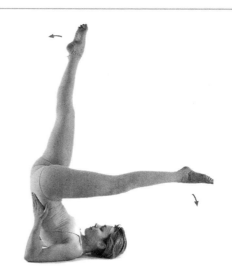

**PREREQUISITES:** The Hundreds: Alternating Legs (Exercise 31), Roll-Over: Bent Legs (Exercise 61), Jackknife (Exercise 65).

**PURPOSE:** To increase abdominal control, stretch the upper back and neck, mobilize the hips, and stretch the hip flexors.

### EXERCISE DESCRIPTION:

*Starting Position:* Lie on your back with your legs extended, hands by your sides, palms down.

a) Engage the B-Line Core and ocean breathe out to do a jackknife (Exercise 65) to the ceiling. In the vertical position, place your hands on the small of your back to support your hips in an upright position; keep the elbows pressed into the mat and close to each other.

b) Keeping the knees locked, toes pointed, and buttocks firmly contracted, ocean breathe out to stretch the right leg toward the floor in the direction of your buttocks, moving the foot past an imaginary line extending vertically from where the elbows rest on the floor. At the same time, lower and stretch the left leg over your head so that the left knee is in line with your eyes (see figure).

c) Breathe in to bring both legs to the vertical position, squeezing the inner thighs together, and smoothly change legs.

d) Ocean breathe out to repeat step b) using the opposite legs.

### KEY POINTS:

1. As the leg stretches up past the imaginary line extending upward from the elbows, draw the hipbones away from the rib cage.

2. A triangle of your hands, elbows, and shoulders provides the foundation for the movement. The control always comes firmly from the B-Line Core.

3. Keep the neck relaxed and lengthened.

4. The hands should be lightly supporting the lower back, not providing the main support.

5. The chin should be slightly off the chest so the breathing can flow easily.

**REPETITIONS:** One set of five on each side.

**BREATHING REVIEW:** Ocean breathe out on the scissors. Breathe in on the close of the legs.

**INCREASE THE CHALLENGE:** Perform the scissors more rapidly. Breathe in for two scissors and ocean breathe out for two scissors: in, in (stretch, stretch), out, out (stretch, stretch).

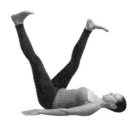

**REDUCE THE CHALLENGE:** Perform the entire exercise with the hips on the floor, head on a flat cushion and hands by the sides, palms down and away from the sides of the body. Start with the legs straight and extended upward directly over the hips, at a ninety-degree angle to the floor.

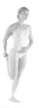

# Bicycle

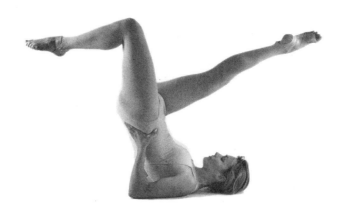

**PREREQUISITE:** Scissors (Exercise 66).

**PURPOSE:** To mobilize the hip joints, keep the abdominals long and strong, stretch the hip flexors, and stabilize the pelvic area.

### EXERCISE DESCRIPTION:

*Starting Position:* The starting position is the same as for the Scissors. Once you have attained the upright position, go on to the following steps:

a) Engage the B-Line Core and ocean breathe out to extend the left leg toward the floor in the direction of your buttocks, taking it past the imaginary line extending vertically from the elbows. At the same time bend the left knee, reaching the toes toward the floor (see figure).

b) Breathe in to now draw the left knee over the head, straightening the leg and extending it toward the ceiling, with the knee above the eyes. At the same time lower the right leg toward the floor in the direction of the buttocks, past the vertical line extending from the elbows. Bend the right knee and extend the toes toward the floor.
  The action is like that of pedaling a bicycle (hence, the name of the exercise).

### KEY POINTS:

1. When you bend the knee to point the toes to the floor in the direction of your buttocks, consciously stretch the front of the thigh as you extend the leg.

2. Imagine the area from the hip to the rib being stretched.

3. As the knee straightens and lengthens over the head above the eyes, squeeze the Core.

4. Do not draw the knee toward the face or chest; keep the cycling action away from the chest.

5. As the foot extends toward the floor, keep any excessive pressure off the hands in order to avoid placing more pressure on the lower back.

**REPETITIONS:** One set of five cycling motions with each leg.

**BREATHING REVIEW:** Ocean breathe out to stretch the leg toward the floor. Breathe in for the cycle movement.

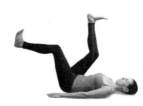

**REDUCE THE CHALLENGE:** Perform the entire exercise with the hips on the floor, head on a flat cushion and hands by the sides, palms down and away from the sides of the body. Start with the legs straight and extended upward directly over the hips, at a ninety-degree angle to the floor. Now start the cycling action with the legs above the B-Line Core.

# Shoulder Bridge

**PREREQUISITE:** The Hundreds: Alternating Legs (Exercise 31), Thigh Stretches (Exercises 11 through 13).

**PURPOSE:** To extend and strengthen the lower back while providing support for the abdominals, and to stretch the hip flexors.

### EXERCISE DESCRIPTION:

*Starting Position:* Lie on your back with the knees bent, feet flat on the floor and parallel, hands by your sides, palms down, and with your neck lengthened. Decompress the spine.

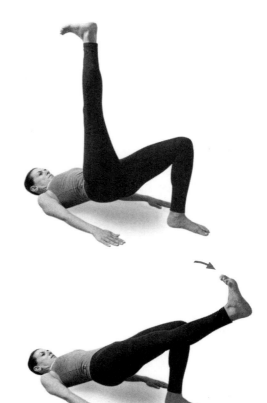

a) Engage the B-Line Core and ocean breathe out to tuck the pelvis and curl the hips up from the mat, lengthening the neck. Press your pelvis to the ceiling, keeping your shoulders, hips, and knees in a straight line.

b) Breathe in to point the right foot and extend the leg straight up to the ceiling, directly above the hip.

c) Ocean breathe out to flex the foot and slowly lower the leg to the floor. Press the heel as far as you can toward the ground, keeping the hips immobile. To prevent the hips from lowering, imagine that you are arching them over a ball.

d) Point the foot and breathe in to quickly kick through the stretched right toe as high and as far back above the head as you can. Then flex the foot and repeat the kick with the same leg.

### KEY POINTS:

1. The shoulders, elbows, and feet support the position.

2. Squeeze the B-Line Core.

3. When lowering the leg, stretch the top of the thigh, "zip up" the stomach, and imagine you are tucking the pelvis under to open the lower back.

4. Keep the lower back as open as possible, especially when the leg lowers to the floor.

5. If you feel the hamstring in your supporting leg cramping, try flexing the foot or moving it farther away.

**REPETITIONS:** Five kicks with the right leg, five kicks with the left.

**BREATHING REVIEW:** Ocean breathe out to lower the leg and stretch it toward the floor. Breathe in to kick up to the ceiling.

**INCREASE THE CHALLENGE:** Place the hands under the hips as in Bicycle (Exercise 67). If there is too much pressure on the wrists, turn the fingers to face outward.

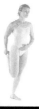

# Can-Can

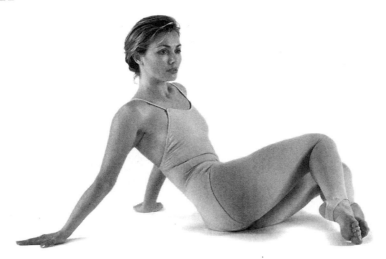

**PREREQUISITES:** The Hundreds: Alternating Legs (Exercise 31), Side to Side (Exercise 23).

**PURPOSE:** To mobilize the lower back and hips, and to activate the obliques.

### EXERCISE DESCRIPTION:

*Starting Position:* Sit upright with your hands behind you on the floor, elbows straight. Place your feet close to your buttocks, with the toes pointed and touching the floor. Keep the knees together.

a) Engage the B-Line Core and ocean breathe out to lower both knees to the left toward the floor, keeping the top of the knees in line with each other. The right buttock and toes will lift off the floor.

b) Squeeze the Core more firmly and, flattening the ribs, breathe in to raise both knees back to the starting position by drawing the left hip toward the right rib cage.

c) Repeat to the other side, gradually lowering the knees closer to the floor each time.

### KEY POINTS:

1. Keep the shoulders and upper torso as still as possible.

2. On each movement to the side, feel the lower back on that side opening. Squeeze the inner thighs together.

3. Lengthen through the crown of the head, drawing the shoulder blades into the pocket.

4. You will feel as if you are walking forward on your buttocks. To counteract this action, walk backward when drawing the knees back to the center.

5. If you feel any twinge or strain in the lower back, do not lower the knees as far.

**REPETITIONS:** Ten repetitions on each side.

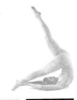

# Can-Can Extension

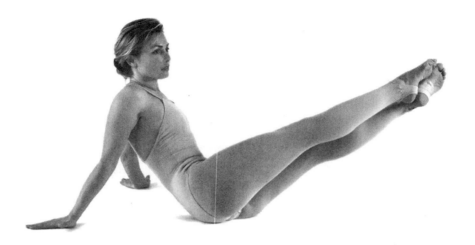

PREREQUISITE: Can-Can (Exercise 69-1).

PURPOSE: To mobilize and strengthen the lower back, hips, and lower abdominals.

EXERCISE DESCRIPTION: This is the advanced version of the Can-Can.

*Starting Position:* As in the Can-Can.

a) Engage the B-Line Core and, after breathing out to lower the knees to the side (less than you did for the Can-Can), breathe in to then extend the legs into the air, still keeping them together and drawing the knees toward your shoulder.

b) Ocean breathe out to draw the heels back to your tailbone, and continue as you did for the Can-Can to the other side.

### KEY POINTS:

1. Avoid leaning back as the legs extend. Lift the ribs toward the knees.

2. Keep the arms and back as straight as possible.

3. At first, the thighs may feel as if they are gripping during the extension, but this will gradually ease.

4. Stop at a comfortable number of repetitions if you are unable to complete ten.

REPETITIONS: Ten on each side.

*Notes*

...........................................................

...........................................................

...........................................................

...........................................................

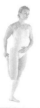

# Hip Circles

*This is similar to the advanced Corkscrew, but it is done in a seated position.*

**PREREQUISITES:** Corkscrew 2: Advanced (Exercise 47-3), Pendulum (Exercise 62), Can-Can Extension (Exercise 69-2).

**PURPOSE:** To increase abdominal and hip-flexor strength, hip-joint mobility, and lower-back mobility.

### EXERCISE DESCRIPTION:

*Starting Position:* Sit upright on the mat. Engage the B-Line Core. Keeping your spine as straight as possible, lean back with your hands behind you so the arms are at a forty-five-degree angle to the floor. Keep the hands wide apart and the elbows straight (but not hyperextended).

a) Breathe in to draw your knees to your chest, and then extend them toward the ceiling, with the feet pointed. Squeeze the inner thighs together.

b) Ocean breathe out to swing the legs around in a circle to the right, lowering them to just off the mat, and then around to the left.

c) Breathe in to squeeze the inner thighs together and stretch the toes toward the ceiling, drawing the knees to the shoulder and then back to the center, and keeping the thighs as close to your chest as possible. Lift the ribs toward the knees to lift out of the lower back.

d) Repeat in the other direction.

### KEY POINTS:

1. Lengthen the neck out of the shoulders, and keep the shoulder blades drawn into the pocket.

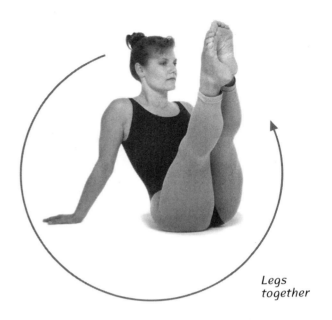

*Legs together*

2. Keep the chest open, and maintain the B-Line Core at all times.

3. Scoop the stomach to raise the legs upward.

4. Keep the hips as square as you can. The hips will slightly rise off the floor as you lower your legs to the sides.

5. As the legs lower to the floor, flatten the ribs toward the hips, keeping the spine long. Lengthen through the toes.

6. If you feel a strain in the wrists or shoulders do the "Reduce the Challenge" version.

**REPETITIONS:** Up to five Hip Circles in each direction.

**BREATHING REVIEW:** Ocean breathe out on the lower part of the circle. Breathe in to raise the legs toward the ceiling.

**REDUCE THE CHALLENGE:** Perform the entire exercise while leaning back on the elbows. The legs will lift higher toward the ceiling, and the gripping of the quads will be reduced. Keep the eyes to the ceiling and the shoulder blades drawn into the pocket.

# Lying Torso Stretch

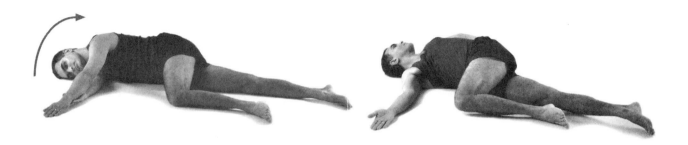

**PREREQUISITE:** Side to Side (Exercise 23).

**PURPOSE:** This is a cooling-down stretch. It mobilizes the middle and upper back and shoulders and releases tension in the lower back.

### EXERCISE DESCRIPTION:

*Starting Position:* Lying on your right side, straighten the right leg and bend the left leg so the left knee and foot are resting on the floor in front of you, with the left heel touching the right knee. Lengthen the right arm in front of the chest, with the palm up. Place a cushion under the head for more comfort. Stretch the left arm in front of the chest, reaching as far as possible through the fingertips, past the right hand; lean the left shoulder forward.

a) Engage the B-Line Core and breathe in to graze the floor with the fingers of the left hand, making a semicircle until the arm is above the head.

b) Ocean breathe out to complete the circle, taking the left arm behind the body, palm upward, and turning the head to face the ceiling. Turn the left shoulder backward to face the ceiling and open the left armpit to the ceiling. Keep the left knee pressed into the ground.

c) Complete the circle by taking the left hand toward the right foot and forward in front of the chest to the starting position.

### KEY POINTS:

1. As the shoulder loosens and the upper back becomes more flexible, the circling hand may eventually touch the floor for the movement.

2. As the arm extends behind the body, lengthen the entire body from the toes of the lower leg through the fingertips of the circling arm.

3. If the muscles feel tight during a particular point of the stretch, stay in that position for several seconds to release the tension before continuing.

4. Do not force the top shoulder down to the floor. Allow the body to release into the stretch gradually.

5. Keep the breathing nice and deep.

**REPETITIONS:** One set of ten repetitions of five circles on each side.

# Stamina Stretch: Advanced

Add the following after the final step in Exercise 2-2: Place the left (outside) leg behind the right leg, and rest it on the outside edge of the left heel. Bend the right leg and continue as for Exercise 2-2. This will add a greater stretch for the top of the outside hip and a mild stretch for the TFL (tensor fasciae latae).

*Notes*

...................................................

...................................................

...................................................

...................................................

...................................................

...................................................

...................................................

...................................................

...................................................

...................................................

...................................................

...................................................

...................................................

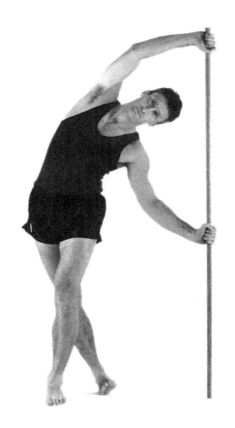

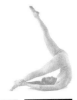

# Lumbar Stretch

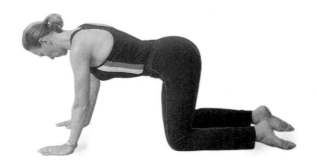 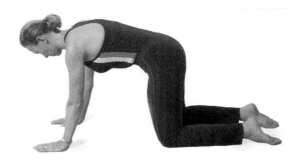

**PREREQUISITE:** None.

**PURPOSE:** To increase flexion mobility of the tight lower spine.

### EXERCISE DESCRIPTION:

*Starting Position:* Kneel on all fours, with the knees and hands shoulder distance apart. Relax the head in line with the spine.

a) Ocean breathe out to slowly tuck the pelvis, drawing the B-Line toward the ceiling. Keep the head straight without hunching the shoulders.

b) Breathe in to release until the spine is horizontal to the floor. Lengthen the hips away from the ribs.

### KEY POINTS:

1. Beware of hunching the shoulders, a poor posture observed by most people during their daily activities.

2. Keep the upper spine in a straight line at all times.

3. This exercise is great for pregnant women and for women suffering from menstrual cramps, as it stretches the tight lower-back muscles.

**REPETITIONS:** Ten stretches.

**INCREASE THE CHALLENGE:** When releasing to return to the horizontal, keep squeezing the Core strongly and allow the back to arch toward the floor, without releasing so far that the abdominals hang. This movement strengthens the back muscles. Do not arch the neck excessively—only a slight lift of the chin is great!

# Rocking

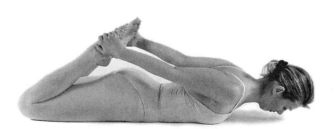

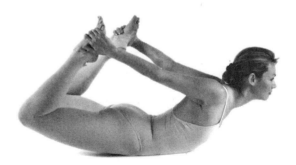

**PREREQUISITES:** Thigh Stretches (Exercises 11 through 13), Swan Dive 2 (Exercise 42-2). *A strong, flexible back is required!*

**PURPOSE:** To control and stretch the front (anterior) part of the torso, and to work and strengthen the back muscles.

### EXERCISE DESCRIPTION:

*Starting Position:* Lie prone (on your stomach) on the mat. Draw your heels to your buttocks and move the knees shoulder width apart, with the feet slightly closer together. Reach behind you and hold the outsides of the feet with your hands. Keep the shoulder blades pressed into the pocket.

a) Strongly engage the B-Line Core, and ocean breathe out to roll forward onto the chest, keeping your chin off the floor and lifting the heels toward the wall above your head.

b) Breathe in to rock backward as hard as you can by pressing the feet toward the wall behind you, opening the chest and lifting it off the mat.

c) Ocean breathe out to rock forward again. Continue the rocking movement.

### KEY POINTS:

1. Think of your spine as the rockers of a rocking chair. As you rock, elongate through the tips of the knees and the crown of the head.

2. Keep the spine as long and open as possible.

3. Keep the abdominals hollow and firm.

4. Keep the shoulder blades drawn into the pocket.

5. Place a pad under the groin if you feel any pressure.

6. If the back feels any pressure, do the "Reduce the Challenge" version.

**REPETITIONS:** One set of up to eight rocking movements.

**BREATHING REVIEW:** Ocean breathe out to roll forward. Breathe in to roll up onto the thighs.

**REDUCE THE CHALLENGE:** Perform the entire exercise by simply breathing in to lift the head and feet toward the ceiling and then breathing out to release back toward the floor by about 90 percent, keeping the B-Line Core engaged at all times.

# Twist 1

**PREREQUISITES:** Hamstring Stretch 3 (Exercise 10), Pendulum (Exercise 62).

**PURPOSE:** To increase rotation of the spine, open the lower back, and mobilize and strengthen the shoulder girdle.

**EXERCISE DESCRIPTION:**

*Starting Position:* Sit partially on your right hip, knees toward the chest, left ankle over the right. Place the sole of the left foot flat on the mat, toes pointing forward, heels close to the tailbone. Place the right hand close to the right hip, with the palm pressed into the mat and fingers pointed forward. Lean slightly forward over the hand. Relax the left hand on the left ankle.

a) Engage the B-Line Core and breathe in to lift your tailbone toward the ceiling as if you were being lifted by a piece of string attached to it. The balance control comes from the palm of the right hand and the sole of the left foot.

b) As the tailbone extends upward, circle the left arm away from the body in a smooth arc up toward the ceiling and over toward the floor close to the left ear, reaching through the fingertips. The crown of the head and the fingers of the left hand should be reaching toward the mat. Draw the chest to the thighs, and look at your knees.

c) Ocean breathe out to reverse the movement, squeezing the Core as if you were still being pulled by the tailbone to the ceiling. Extend the left arm to the outside of the thigh as if you were drawing a line with your fingertips along the ceiling and then downward.

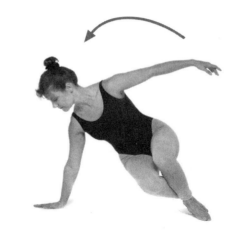
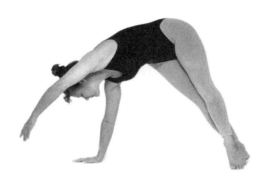

**KEY POINTS:**

1. Keeping the elbow joint unlocked, reach outward through the fingers of the moving arm, as if you were trying to touch the ceiling in both directions.

2. Lift the tailbone as high as you can, trying to straighten the spine and keeping the abdominals hollow. Think also of lifting the B-Line toward the ceiling.

3. Keep the shoulder blades in line with the hips.

4. To achieve balance, place equal pressure on the heel and fingertips of the right hand.

**REPETITIONS:** One set of five on each side.

**BREATHING REVIEW:** Breathe in on the extension to the ceiling. Ocean breathe out on the return to the mat.

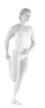

# Twist 2

**PREREQUISITE:** Twist 1 (Exercise 75-1).

**PURPOSE:** To achieve advanced balance and control.

**EXERCISE DESCRIPTION:**

*Starting Position:* Sit upright on the mat, legs extended in front of you; place your right hand on the floor slightly behind you, and lean over onto the right hip so that your torso faces away from the upright position. Cross the left leg on top of the right leg. Relax the left hand on the floor in front of the thigh (Figure i).

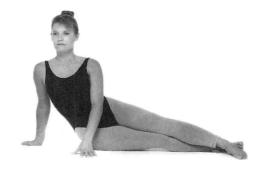

*Figure i*

a) Engage the B-Line Core and breathe in to lift the left hipbone vertically as if it were attached to a string drawing upward. The control comes from pressing the sole of the left foot into the floor as much as possible. Squeeze the inner thighs together.

b) As the movement begins, extend the left hand (elbow unlocked) toward the left foot, then draw a line to the ceiling and over toward a point above the left ear. Maintain absolute control (Figure ii).

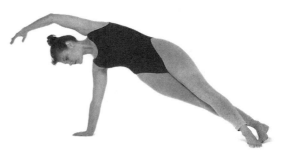

*Figure ii*

c) Ocean breathe out to rotate only the torso to face the floor by rotating the left shoulder blade toward the right hand and tucking the left hand under the body and past the right armpit. Feel the obliques on both sides connect. Keep the left arm in line with the ear and the left shoulder blade drawn toward the left hip.

d) Breathe in to rotate the torso back as if you were opening your chest to the ceiling, sweeping the left hand out from under the body to the side wall, then upward as far as possible, as if you were drawing a line along the ceiling. The obliques and the Core are still strongly engaged. Stretch the top of the thighs (Figure iii).

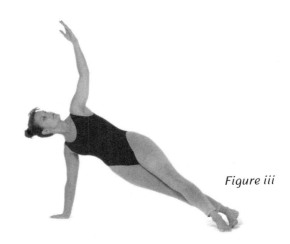

*Figure iii*

# Twist 2 *(cont'd.)*

e) Ocean breathe out to return to the starting position, reversing the movements in steps b and a.

### KEY POINTS:

1. When lifting the hip to the ceiling you should achieve a straight line, as if along a pole, from the feet, to the tailbone, through the spine, and to the crown of the head.

2. Keep the pelvis tucked under for better lower-abdominal connection (this is not usually visually apparent; it is the internal connection that is more important).

3. Maintain careful, smooth control during the rotation of the torso. It is a precise movement that requires every fiber of the body to be active and all your concentration to be focused for the best result.

**REPETITIONS:** One set of up to five Twists on each side.

**BREATHING REVIEW:** Breathe in on the lift. Ocean breathe out to rotate toward the floor and breathe in to rotate toward the ceiling. Ocean breathe out to return to the starting position.

*Notes*

........................................

........................................

........................................

........................................

........................................

........................................

........................................

........................................

........................................

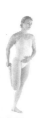

# 10

# MORE CHALLENGING EXERCISES

When all
your muscles
are properly
developed, you
will, as a matter
of course, perform
your work with
minimum effort
and maximum
pleasure.

— J. PILATES

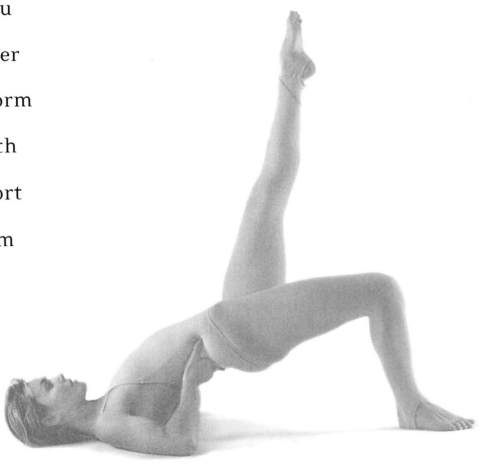

# Oblique Curls

**PREREQUISITE:** The Perfect Abdominal Curl (Exercise 25).

**PURPOSE:** An advanced exercise to strengthen the obliques.

**EXERCISE DESCRIPTION:** In essence, this exercise is the same as the Curl but with a twist.

*Starting Position:* Lie on your back with your feet on the floor, knees bent in a right angle. Engage the B-Line Core and contract forward with the fingers interlocked behind the head and the elbows open.

   a) Ocean breathe out to draw the right armpit toward the left knee, keeping the elbows open. Imagine you have a golf ball under your chin so you do not pull the head forward and strain the neck. Scoop the stomach.

   b) Breathe in to scoop the abdominals and release the torso until the shoulder blades almost touch the floor.

   c) Smoothly roll across the middle part of the back to the other side, and repeat.

**KEY POINTS:**

1. Keep the shoulder blades lifted off the floor at all times.

2. Keep the elbows open wide so there is less strain on the neck.

3. Turn the head and shoulders and look to the side for maximum rotation of the torso (where the eyes go, the body follows).

4. Keep the hips still, planted into the mat. Maintain the B-Line Core at all times.

5. *Turn and lift* the torso each time.

**REPETITIONS:** One set of ten on each side.

*Notes*

# Wrist and Forearm Strengthener

**PREREQUISITE:** None.

**PURPOSE:** To strengthen the wrists and forearms for all racquet sports and other sports that require finger or wrist strength.

**EXERCISE DESCRIPTION:** Get a piece of thin rope approximately five feet long. Drill a hole through a wooden pole (twelve inches long), pass the rope through the hole, and tie a knot at one end. At the other end of the rope, tie a weight of four to eight pounds or a bag of sand.

*Starting Position:* Stand up and engage the B-Line Core. Hold the pole at shoulder height in front of you, arms extended. If the weight is resting on the floor, make the rope shorter.

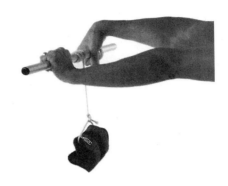

a) Always keeping a firm hold on the pole so that it doesn't slide through the fingers or palm, slowly open the palm of the right hand and turn the wrist back to take hold of the underside of the pole. Grip the pole and rotate the right wrist forward as far as possible so that the knuckles are pointing toward the floor.

b) At the same time, turn the left wrist back and grip the pole. Now extend the left wrist forward as far as possible.

c) Keep repeating this movement, taking both wrists through the extreme ranges of forward and backward motion until the rope has wound all the way up the pole. There should be enough pole for the rope to roll onto without hindering the hands' grip. Breathe deeply, closing the rib cage on every breath out.

d) Once the rope is totally rolled up, reverse the wrist movement so you unroll the weight down to the floor. Again, do not let the pole slide through the fingers.

e) When the rope is unrolled, do not stop. Continue the unrolling action of the wrist so the rope once again begins to wind onto the pole. Repeat the movement up and down three times.

### KEY POINTS:

1. At the end of the exercise, the muscles in the forearm may feel as if they will burst through the skin because they are so pumped up!

2. Rotate the wrists forward and backward as fully as possible.

3. Keep the pole parallel to the floor throughout the exercise.

4. Vary the weight according to your requirements and strength. This exercise is a challenge!

5. Do as many complete rolls of the rope up and down as possible. At first, you may only be able to go up and down once. Aim for three times up and down.

6. Keep the shoulder blades drawn into the pocket. Do not lean backward.

For those with weaker shoulders, the exercise can be done with the elbows by the sides and the forearms horizontal to the floor. Work toward performing the exercise with the arms extended at shoulder level.

# Neck Stretches

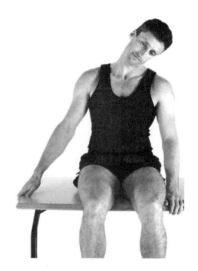

*Figure i*

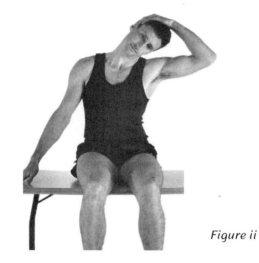

*Figure ii*

**PREREQUISITE:** A tight neck!

**PURPOSE:** To loosen tight neck muscles.

### EXERCISE DESCRIPTION:

*Starting Position:* Sit upright on a chair or on a bench on your sitz bones (Figure i). Plant the feet on the floor hip distance apart. With the right hand, hold firmly onto the bench or onto the back leg of the chair.

    a) Ocean breathe out to stretch the left ear toward the left shoulder, pressing both shoulder blades toward the hips. You should feel the stretch strongly on the right side of the neck. Take a breath in.

    b) Now ocean breathe out to turn the head slightly toward the ceiling. You should feel the stretch more toward the front of the neck.

### KEY POINTS:

1. The stretch should be mild at the beginning.

2. Continue only if the stretch feels good.

3. If you feel any discomfort in the neck, stop the exercise.

**REPETITIONS:** Six to ten breaths in and out for each direction (right and left).

**INCREASE THE CHALLENGE:** You can obtain a stronger stretch by placing the opposite hand on the top of the head and slightly toward the ear of the side being stretched (Figure ii).

    Breathe out to press the head against the pressure of the hand without allowing the head to move. This isometric stretch will allow the neck muscles to lengthen further. Do not pull the head toward the floor!

Breathe in to allow the head to relax further before repeating. Press the shoulder of the side being stretched firmly toward the floor. The resistance from the hand on the head should be no more than 50 percent to start with.

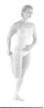

# Seated Spine Rotation

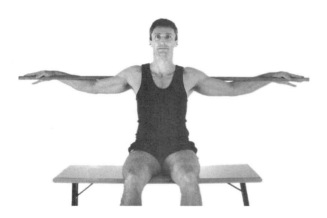

*Figure i*

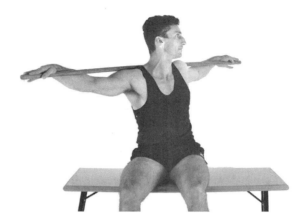

*Figure ii*

**PREREQUISITE:** Side to Side (Exercise 23), Corkscrew 2: Advanced (Exercise 47-3) or Pendulum (Exercise 62).

**PURPOSE:** To stretch the tight muscles of the spine and obliques, and to increase rotational mobility.

### EXERCISE DESCRIPTION:

*Starting Position:* Sit upright on a chair or on a bench on your sitz bones with a slight pelvic tuck so the spine is straight (Figure i). Plant the feet on the floor hip distance apart. Place a long pole across the back of the shoulders parallel to the floor, and lengthen the arms along the pole with the hands holding on to the top of it.

  a) Engage the B-Line Core. Ocean breathe out to stretch the left shoulder to a point behind you, keeping the arms horizontal and pressing both shoulders toward the floor. Look over your shoulder. Grow taller as you turn.

  b) Squeeze the Core and breathe in to rotate the torso back to the center.

  c) Without stopping, repeat to the other side.

### KEY POINTS:

1. The stretch should be mild at the beginning. Continue only if the stretch feels good.

2. Turn the head around as much as you can without straining the neck: where the eyes go, the body follows.

3. Keep the pole parallel to the floor at all times.

4. Keep the shoulder blades pressed into the pocket.

5. Keep the hips square at all times; press through the knee of the side to which you are turning.

6. If you feel any discomfort in the back, shoulders, or neck, stop the exercise.

**REPETITIONS:** Ten to each side. Once you are proficient with the exercise, you can speed up the movement.

# Cushion Squeeze

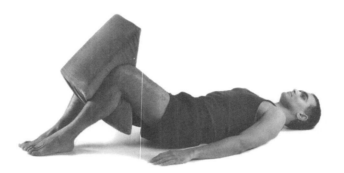

**PREREQUISITE:** None.

**PURPOSE:** To strengthen and tone the inner thighs (adductors).

### EXERCISE DESCRIPTION:

*Starting Position:* Lie on your back on the floor with the knees bent and the feet flat on the floor about twelve inches apart. Place a firm cushion or several pillows between the knees.

a) Engage the B-Line Core, and ocean breathe out to squeeze the cushion between the thighs. Maintain the Stable Spine position, and avoid squeezing the buttocks.

b) Breathe in to release about 10 percent of the squeeze before repeating.

**KEY POINTS:**

1. The squeeze should be mild at the beginning. Gradually keep squeezing harder.

2. If you feel this in the muscles near the groin, stop. You should feel the exercise only in the inner thighs, a short distance away from the groin.

3. To make the exercise even more effective, turn the toes inward and feel the difference!

4. The exercise can also be done with abdominal curls: curl up on the squeeze.

**REPETITIONS:** Two sets of ten squeezes, with a fifteen-second rest between each set.

*Notes*

. . . . . . . . . . . . . . . . . . . . . . . . . . . . . . . . . . . . . . . . . . . . . . . . . . . . . . . . . . .

. . . . . . . . . . . . . . . . . . . . . . . . . . . . . . . . . . . . . . . . . . . . . . . . . . . . . . . . . . .

. . . . . . . . . . . . . . . . . . . . . . . . . . . . . . . . . . . . . . . . . . . . . . . . . . . . . . . . . . .

. . . . . . . . . . . . . . . . . . . . . . . . . . . . . . . . . . . . . . . . . . . . . . . . . . . . . . . . . . .

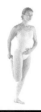

# 11

# Theraband Routines

Be certain

that you have

your entire body

under complete

mental control.

— J. Pilates

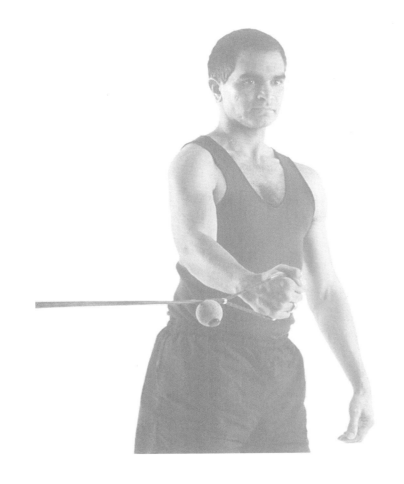

The following series of exercises is done with a Theraband or similar wide elastic band. An Australian product called the IsoToner is particularly useful as it comes with a handle and cork balls for a better grip, as well as a piece of rope for locking into a door or tying to a door handle. (Please see the ad at the end of the book for information on purchasing the IsoToner product illustrated in these exercises.)

There are no prerequisite exercises for this series, and anyone should be able to manage the exercises comfortably as the IsoToner comes in various strengths. There is a suitable resistance for everyone.

The photographs are straightforward and clearly illustrate the movements required. All of these exercises involve doing one or two sets of ten repetitions per side.

**CAUTION:** *Never pull the Theraband directly into your face.*

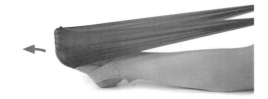

## Exercise TB 1:

### Pointing the Foot (Plantar Flexion)

This exercise strengthens the calf muscles, the intrinsic muscles of the foot, and the ankle joint. Make sure that the toe is kept in line with the knee, and not sickling inward. Using the muscles of the feet, press through the ball of the toe, at the same time stretching the top of the foot. These muscles are necessary for jumping, rising onto the ball of the foot, and balancing on the ball of the foot.

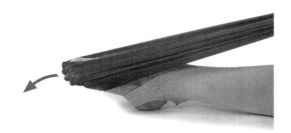

## Exercise TB 2:

### Pointing the Toes

This exercise strengthens the smaller muscles and tendons in the bottom of the foot, which are important for strengthening the toes. After you've extended through the ball of the foot, work only on flexion and extension of the toes, without flexing the foot at the ankle (that is, keep the foot extended in a "pointed" position). Do not crunch the toes when extending. For ballet dancers, this is necessary for pointe work, jumping, and developing a pleasing line of the foot.

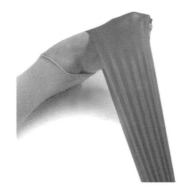

## Exercise TB 3:

### Dorsiflexion of the Ankle

Support the working foot by resting it on the bent knee of the opposite leg. Keep the foot pointed and apply pressure from the IsoToner. Draw the foot inward toward the knee of the same leg, working the muscles and tendon on the top of the foot. This strengthens the front of the ankle and the muscles on the outside (lateral side) of the calf to provide ankle support. Dorsiflexion is necessary when landing from a jump.

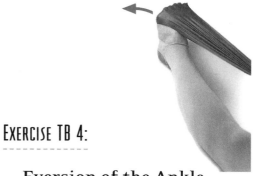

## Exercise TB 4:

### Eversion of the Ankle

This exercise strengthens the muscles surrounding the ankle and the muscles on the lateral side (outside) of the calf. Still pointing the toes, and while applying gentle opposing pressure from the IsoToner, work on straightening the foot from a turned-in or inverted position. This strengthening will help prevent ankle sprains as well as aid their speedy recovery. It also helps in stabilizing the ankle joint on flat surfaces or when rising onto the toe. For dancers, this strength is important in preventing "sickling" of the foot.

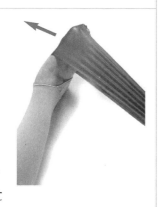

## Exercise TB 5:

### Inversion of the Metatarsal Joint

This exercise will develop muscles in the front (anterior) part of the lower leg along the shin bone, as well as in the arch of the foot. Start with the foot pointed and the resistance of the IsoToner attempting to draw the foot in an outward direction. Still lengthening through the toes, "curl" the arch of the foot inward to strengthen the inside muscle groups. This is necessary in stabilizing the muscles of the ankle and will help prevent the rolling in of the foot.

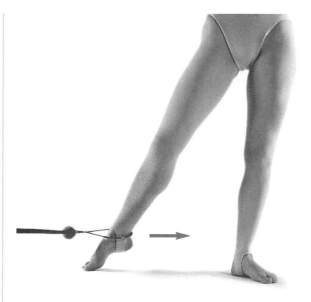

## Exercise TB 6:

### Adduction of the Inner Thigh

Place the rope end of the IsoToner in a door at calf level and close the door with the loop on the other side of the door. This will hold the IsoToner securely. This exercise strengthens the inner thigh muscles (adductors) of both the working leg and the supporting leg. Turn out the working leg with the IsoToner wrapped around the ankle, and draw the heel toward the supporting foot. Keep the knees of both the working leg and the supporting leg straight (but not locked). The muscle that is actually worked is in the top of the inner thigh. As you release the foot, point it, keeping tension in the IsoToner. For ballet dancers, this exercise develops the stability of the standing leg, helps build speed for *petite allegro,* and is necessary for *batterie (cabrioles, entrechat six, entrechat huit,* switching legs in *double tours,* etc.).

## Exercise TB 7:

### Flexion and Extension of the Leg while Using Outward Rotation of the Hip Joints

This is another exercise to strengthen the inner thigh muscles of both legs. It helps greatly with the external rotation of the thigh (femur). If you feel any discomfort in the knee joint, bend the knee slightly. Start with both legs together and extend the working foot forward as far as possible, pointing the foot at the same time, then returning to the starting position. Be sure to keep the working leg slightly turned out from the hip; think of leading the movement with the inner thigh rather than with the front of the leg.

## Exercise TB 8:

### Hyperextension to Extension

This exercise is designed to strengthen the front of the inner thigh. The resistance required to bring the leg from the hyperextended position (behind you) to the extended position (legs together) is helpful in working the muscles around and, especially, in the front of othe hip socket. Perform the exercise without arching the back when the leg hyperextends (engaging the B-Line Core will help a great deal). Keep the working leg turned out from the hip; think of leading the movement with the inside of the leg rather than with the front of the leg.

## Exercise TB 9:

### Flexion to Extension on the Back

Place the loop of the IsoToner over the top of a door and shut the door so the loop is securely fastened. Lie on your back and place one foot in the handle of the IsoToner. Keeping both legs turned out, draw the working leg down to the floor. This movement strengthens and tones the posterior (behind) part of the legs, including the gluteus (buttock) muscles. This strength is required for isolation from the hip joint and stability in the pelvic region (ballet dancers: for jumps and *adagios*).

## Exercise TB 10:

### Prone Hyperextension to Extension

Lying on the stomach, engage the B-Line Core, keep the hipbones flat on the floor, and externally rotate the legs (insides of the legs toward the floor). Now draw the working leg down toward the floor. The resistance will create strength and tone in the front of the thighs.

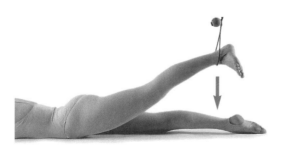

## Exercise TB 11:

### Biceps

Place the rope end of the IsoToner in a door at about calf level and close the door with the loop on the other side of the door. This will hold the IsoToner securely. Hold the handle and sit three to four feet away from the door. Rest the working elbow on the bent knee. Draw the handle to the shoulder, stretching the IsoToner. Resist the tension upon release. Don't allow the wrist to bend either inward or outward. This should feel as if the middle of the forearm is drawing toward the biceps, rather than the hand toward the shoulder.

## Exercise TB 12:

### Triceps

Sit on the floor with your back to the door and about three to four feet away. Rest the working elbow on the bent knee and extend the arm down toward the floor to a fully extended position. Don't allow the wrist to bend either inward or outward. Resist upon the release.

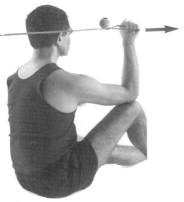

## Exercise TB 13:

### Pectorals

Stand at a ninety-degree angle to the door, about three to six feet away. The band should be positioned in the closed door at about waist level. Hold the handle, and with a slightly flexed (bent) elbow, draw the IsoToner across the chest. Keep the elbow in a fixed position and do not rotate the upper body to move the arm farther. Do not allow the wrist to bend either inward or outward.

## Exercise TB 14:

### Pectorals and Deltoids

Stand with your back to the door, about three to six feet away. Hold the handle and keep the elbow in a flexed (bent) position. Draw the handle forward to the hip and then continue forward to shoulder level. Resist upon the return. Keep the upper body stable. Don't allow the arm to rise upward and away from the body. Don't allow the wrist to bend either inward or outward.

## Exercise TB 15:

### Latissimus Dorsi

Stand at a ninety-degree angle to a closed door, about three to six feet away. Hold the IsoToner taut away from the body, arm straight but not locked. Draw the IsoToner to your side, pressing the arm toward the floor. To better connect the lat, imagine you are squashing an orange under the armpit to press the arm to your side. Resist upon the return. Don't allow the wrist to bend either inward or outward.

## Exercise TB 16:

### Back

Face the door, standing about three to six feet away. With the arm extended forward at chest level, draw the handle in a circular motion as far to the outside as possible. Keep the arm parallel to the floor. Keep the shoulders square to the door at all times. Imagine drawing the shoulder blades together; this will strengthen the rhomboid muscles between the shoulder blades. Don't allow the wrist to bend.

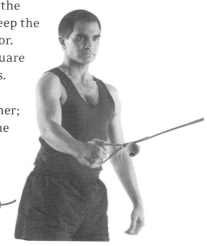

## Exercise TB 17:

### Overhead

Stand at a ninety-degree angle to the door with the working arm extended upward at about a forty-five-degree angle to the door. Keeping a slight bend in the elbow, extend the arm overhead away from the door. Don't allow the wrist to bend. This exercise will work the shoulder muscles. If you feel any discomfort in the neck, stop the exercise.

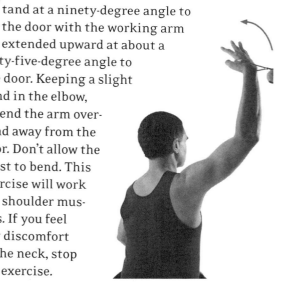

## Exercise TB 18:

### Side Stretch

Stand at a ninety-degree angle to the door. With the IsoToner secured to the bottom of the door, place your free hand on the side of the head, keeping the elbow open wide. Stretch to the side, extending through the tip of the elbow in an arc so the side does not crunch. Lift up and out of the hip as if stretching over a ball. Keep the hips firm and square. This is an important exercise for strengthening the side muscles (quadratus lumborum).

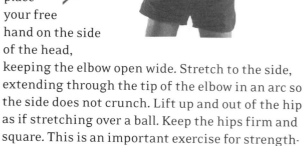

# 12

# MOVE YOURSELF OUT OF PAIN

Physical fitness can neither be acquired by wishful thinking nor by outright purchase. However, it can be gained through performing these (daily) exercises conceived for this purpose by the founder of Contrology whose unique methods accomplish this desirable result by successfully counteracting the harmful, inherent conditions associated with modern civilization.

— FROM *Return to Life Through Contrology*

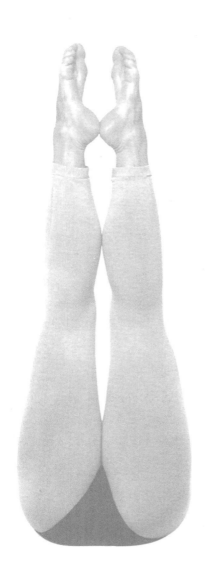

The ultimate goal of any therapeutic or rehabilitation exercise program is to achieve pain-free movement. But many people who are in some pain, even though they have passed the acute stage of their problem, are still reluctant to move the areas of the body where they previously felt pain. This protective attitude toward the body can be detrimental in the long term to a person's well-being.

This mental protection of the physical structure inhibits recovery, rehabilitation, and progress to normal movement. Over time an imbalance is created, which the body will accept as normal, and which the mind eventually also accepts.

In this chapter we will discuss general rehabilitation exercises for the various parts of the body in cases where the condition is no longer in the acute phases and the treating practitioner has given permission for a postacute exercise program.

It is important to realize that beginning an exercise program does not mean immediate relief. Even though some of the benefits may be immediate, and although the mind may be willing to achieve a normal lifestyle, the body is still physically weak. Too often it has been reported that when the symptoms of pain have disappeared for some minutes, the patient assumes that the condition is fixed and that he is able to return to normal activity. Sadly, this is far from the truth. The feeling of well-being may only be temporary. Although the injury may have taken only a matter of seconds to inflict, it may take months to repair. This can be very frustrating to the individual who is on a mission to be better in the shortest time possible. Remember, however, that it was the tortoise who won the race!

The exercise rehabilitation process has two main objectives:

1. To reduce the recovery time for each episode in which the injured area is affected by overexertion, either intentionally or accidentally.

2. To substantially strengthen the area.

Say, for example, an individual has lower-back pain. She has not begun any exercise program;

## SANJAY P.

*Sanjay P., a middle-aged man of slightly larger than average build, had dislocated his right shoulder eight times in the previous two years. Previous rehabilitation exercises involved raising weights, in a standing position, up to shoulder level and no higher.*

*When asked about the mobility of the joint, he responded that he was only able to raise the arm to shoulder height and would not attempt to raise it any higher (possibly for fear of another dislocation), even without weights.*

*The last dislocation had occurred eight months previously; Sanjay P. was convinced that his current range of movement was set for the rest of his life.*

*After doing a series of arm-weight exercises while lying supine on a narrow bench (never lifting above shoulder height), he was then told to lie face down. He was asked to raise the arms out to the sides to bench level and then to return to the starting position. This was well within his perceived comfort zone, and he completed several repetitions easily.*

*After doing several of these movements, still lying on his stomach, Sanjay P. was then asked to raise the left arm to the left ear and to lower the right arm to the right hip, and then to alternate the movement (similar to a marching movement). He accomplished this without any effort or fear. When he raised the right arm to the ear for the third time, he was asked to hold the position and to imagine that he was in an upright position. This came as quite a surprise to him, as the arm was above head height. He was asked to stand and repeat the movement without fear. Once his fear had been overcome, the rehabilitation of his shoulder was more effective and he saw results faster.*

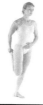

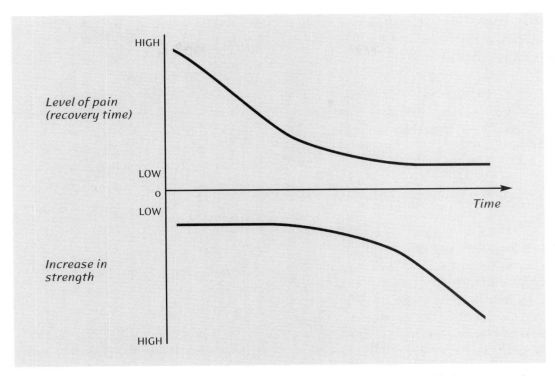

HIGH

Level of pain
(recovery time)

LOW
o
LOW

Time

Increase in
strength

HIGH

*Figure 43.* *The relationship between pain and strength. The relationship between pain and strength is quite apparent. As one experiences higher levels of pain, activity tends to become more restricted and, as a result, muscle strength diminishes. As pain levels decrease and rehabilitative exercise is undertaken, more strength is gained in the muscle groups.*

however, when her back "goes out," it takes two days for the pain to diminish. Starting a personalized exercise program does not mean the problem will be solved overnight. However, if the back goes out again, the program, if effectively implemented, should reduce the recovery time from two days to possibly only a few hours. After that, each time the back goes out, the recovery time should be shorter than it was the last time. As muscular stability is achieved, this recovery time should continue to reduce.

There may be setbacks along the way when the patient will feel more pain. One reason for this is that as the program progresses the imbalance caused by the injury and therefore already accentuated in the patient is exacerbated. This happens because the stronger muscles continue to dominate the movement, while the weaker muscles initially tend to lag behind, producing

further imbalances as the strong muscles "pull" the structure out of alignment. This situation is usually indicated by the fact that discomfort occurs and remains no matter what stretches are prescribed to alleviate it. The discomfort is easily remedied by gentle manipulation to "realign" the problem area, after which the exercise program can be continued. (Please consult your physical therapist if this occurs.)

If you are participating in realignment sessions with a qualified practitioner, it is important to remember that you should do no exercises for at least twenty-four to thirty-six hours after the treatment in order for its effects to settle into the muscular system.

As the recovery time approaches zero, the true strengthening phase of the program can begin. Keep in mind the guidelines mentioned in Chapter 3, under the section "Joint Strains."

## SPECIFIC CONDITIONS AND THE EXERCISES THAT HELP TO RELIEVE THEM

In the descriptions of the conditions that follow, the exercises have been numbered for quick reference but should be performed in the order listed.

### The Ankles and Feet

For weak ankles and feet, including pronation, supination, flat feet, and weak toes:

**All ankle Theraband work:**

| Exercises TB 1 through TB 5 | |
| --- | --- |

**Plus**

| Exercises 8-1, 8-2 | Calf Stretches |
| --- | --- |

### The Knee

For weak knee joints, including chondromalacia of the patella and patella tracking syndrome:

| Exercises 8-1, 8-2 | Calf Stretches |
| --- | --- |
| Exercises 26-1, 26-2, 26-3 | Ankle Weights |

**Plus Theraband:**

| Exercise TB 6 | Adduction of the Inner Thigh |
| --- | --- |
| Exercise TB 8 | Hyperextension to Extension |
| Exercise TB 7 | Flexion and Extension of the Leg while Using Outward Rotation of the Hip Joints |

### The Hip Joint

**Theraband:**

| Exercises TB 6 to TB 10 | |
| --- | --- |

**Plus:**

| Exercise 64 | Helicopter Hundreds |
| --- | --- |
| Exercise 20 | Single Leg Stretch |
| Exercise 22 | Single Leg Circles 1 |
| Exercise 62 | Pendulum |
| Exercise 49 | Side Kick 1 |
| Exercise 56 | Side Kick 2 |
| Exercises 26-1, 26-2, 26-3 | Ankle Weights |
| Exercise 72 | Stamina Stretch: Advanced |

### The Back

Lower-back pain is one of the most common complaints in Western society. The complaints range from minor backache, which can be fixed with massage, manipulation, or anti-inflammatory drugs, to more serious cases, such as disc protrusions and spondylolisthesis (the forward slippage of one vertebra onto another), to those that require surgery.

Clearly graduated exercise programs are the best long-term management for lower-back pain. These take the form of gradual stretching and strengthening.

It is often more important to know what *not* to do, as these movements can set back the program and irritate the condition.

Listed below are some of the movements to *avoid* for certain conditions, followed by simple routines to practice. For all back problems, the start stretches, hamstring stretches, and thigh stretches should be done unless there are contraindications to the stretches.

The following three stretches are to be completed in all cases unless indications are that they are impossible to achieve even in the mildest form:

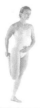

| | |
|---|---|
| Exercises 3 through 6a | The Start Stretches |
| Exercises 9-1, 9-2 | Hamstring Stretches |
| Exercises 11 through 13 | Thigh Stretches (lying, standing, or kneeling, depending on the tightness of the thighs) |

The following basic routine is suggested for most low-grade lower-back pain:

| | |
|---|---|
| Exercise 45 | Spine Stretch |
| Exercise 23 | Side to Side |
| Exercise 18 | The Hundreds: Basic |
| Exercise 32 | Coordination |
| Exercise 21 | Double Leg Stretch: Basic |
| Exercise 20 | Single Leg Stretch |
| Exercise 25 | The Perfect Abdominal Curl |
| Exercise 24 | Stomach Stretch |
| Exercise 51 | Pelvic Curl |
| Exercise 44 | Spine Rotation |
| Exercise 73 | Lumbar Stretch |

For posterior disc bulges, avoid any forward flexion exercises. Instead, do the following:

| | |
|---|---|
| Exercise 24 | Stomach Stretch |
| Exercise 25 | The Perfect Abdominal Curl |
| Exercise 20 | Single Leg Stretch |
| Exercise 21 | Double Leg Stretch: Basic |
| Exercise 22 | Single Leg Circles 1 |
| Exercise 18 | The Hundreds: Basic |

For one-sided sciatic problems, avoid exercises that contract the lower-back muscles on the side where the sciatic pain is located. Stretch the tight side. Follow the exercises below, placing particular emphasis on repeating twice as many sets on the tight side of the back:

| | |
|---|---|
| Exercise 7 | Spiral Stretch |
| Exercise 44 | Spine Rotation |
| Exercise 25 | The Perfect Abdominal Curl |
| Exercise 38 | Crisscross |
| Exercise 50 | Side Leg Lifts |
| Exercise 21 | Double Leg Stretch: Basic |
| Exercise 43 | Swimming |
| Exercise 72 | Stamina Stretch: Advanced |

If you have sciatic pain down both legs, avoid hyperextending the lower back. Follow these exercises:

| | |
|---|---|
| Exercise 51 | Pelvic Curl |
| Exercise 73 | Lumbar Stretch |

If you have scoliosis, avoid leaning the torso toward the short side of the curve. The exercise program is the same as that for one-sided sciatic pain.

If you have lumbar lordosis, avoid arching the back in that area. Follow these exercises:

| | |
|---|---|
| Exercise 2 | Standing Spine Roll |
| Exercise 45 | Spine Stretch |
| Exercise 18 | The Hundreds: Basic |
| Exercise 32 | Coordination |
| Exercise 20 | Single Leg Stretch |
| Exercise 21 | Double Leg Stretch: Basic |
| Exercise 22 | Single Leg Circles 1 |
| Exercise 25 | The Perfect Abdominal Curl |
| Exercise 76 | Oblique Curls |
| Exercise 51 | Pelvic Curl |

## BASIC ROUTINE EXERCISE CHART

| EXERCISE | WEEK 1 | | | WEEK 2 | | | WEEK 3 | | | WEEK 4 | | |
|---|---|---|---|---|---|---|---|---|---|---|---|---|
| PROGRAM DATE: *5 / 17 / 04* | M | W | F | M | W | F | M | W | F | M | W | F |
| #2-1 Standing Roll Down | 7 | 6 | 4 | | | | | | | | | |
| #3 to 6a The Start Stretches | 7 | 6 | 7 | | | | | | | | | |
| #9-1 Hamstring Stretch: Basic | 8 | 8 | 7 | | | | | | | | | |
| #12 Thigh Stretch 2: Standing | 9 | 8 | 7 | | | | | | | | | |
| #45 Spine Stretch | 7 | 7 | 6 | | | | | | | | | |
| #50 Side Leg Lifts | 8 | 8 | 7 | | | | | | | | | |
| #16 Preparation with Cushions | 8 | 7 | 6 | | | | | | | | | |
| #18 The Hundreds: Basic | 8 | 8 | 8 | | | | | | | | | |
| #32 Coordination | 8 | 9 | 8 | | | | | | | | | |
| #20 Single Leg Stretch | 6 | 6 | 6 | | | | | | | | | |
| #21 Double Leg Stretch: Basic | 8 | 7 | 8 | | | | | | | | | |
| #25 The Perfect Abdominal Curl (PAC) | 8 | 8 | 8 | | | | | | | | | |
| #73 Lumbar Stretch | 6 | 6 | 6 | | | | | | | | | |
| #28-2 Opening Arms | 8 | 7 | 7 | | | | | | | | | |
| #29-1, 29-2 Arm Swings | 6 | 6 | 6 | | | | | | | | | |
| #1 Resting Position (Baby Pose) | 8 | 7 | | | | | | | | | | |

*Figure 44. Sample exercise chart*

| Exercise 73 | Lumbar Stretch |
|---|---|
| Exercise 44 | Spine Rotation |
| Exercise 1 | Resting Position (Baby Pose) |

If you have cervical lordosis, lie on the floor and extend the arms at shoulder height away from the body with the palms facing up. Place a small, soft cushion under the arch of the neck and, breathing out, press the neck into the cushion, without rounding the shoulders.

Also do this exercise:

| Exercise 78 | Neck Stretches |
|---|---|

In addition, do the following: Sitting upright, interlock the fingers behind the head. Stretch the chin toward the chest and, breathing out, resist with the hands as you stretch the *back* of the neck toward the ceiling. Do not lift from the top of the head. Press the shoulder blades toward the floor. Repeat ten times.

### The Shoulders

For shoulder problems and kyphosis (middle/upper thoracic spine), avoid forward flexion of the back in that area.

Follow these exercises (always with a cushion under the forehead to support the neck in a stretched position):

| Exercise 39 | Stomach Stretch: Alternating Arms and Legs |
|---|---|
| Exercise 43 | Swimming |
| Exercise 30 | The Pole |
| Exercises 28-2 through 28-5 | Arm Weights |
| Exercises 29-1, 29-2 | Arm Swings |
| Exercise 78 | Neck Stretches |

As an exercise becomes less of a challenge, progress to the next version of the exercise, keeping in mind all the finer points of the exercise listed under Key Points.

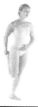

## INCREASING THE CHALLENGE: A PLAN FOR PROGRESSING THROUGH THE EXERCISES

To help you advance through the exercises, I have compiled below several lists of exercises in progressive order. You should begin with the Basic Routine and continue in order through Stage VI. As you progress, bear in mind that the challenge is to control the manner in which you perform the routine, not how many exercises you can do in the shortest period of time.

The Basic Routine is adequate for beginners of any age, including children (if your child is experiencing a growth spurt, first check with your medical practitioner or a qualified Pilates practitioner).

Although the Pilates method has become widely known as an aid in rehabilitating people with many types of injuries and conditions, the various plans presented here do not take into account specific injuries or unusual conditions. Therefore, you should not attempt to use them for rehabilitative purposes without first consulting a qualified health practitioner or Pilates practitioner.

For the convenience of those wishing to record their progress while advancing through the various stages of the program, I have included charts at the end of the book covering the Basic Routine plus Stages I through VI. Or you may purchase the Pilates Personal Training Diary offered at the end of this book. Complete one stage at a time, performing the exercises in the order presented below. Do the exercises three times a week (or more often if you wish). On the chart, in the applicable box for each exercise and date, record the level of effort or challenge you experienced when doing the exercise. Use as your guide the stretch scale and the work scale described in Chapter 3. For example, the following chart shows that on Monday the Standing Spine Roll required an effort of 7 out of 10. If the challenge falls below 6 out of 10, then progress to a harder version of the exercise. If there isn't a harder version, then progress to a different but similar exercise that poses a challenge. (It may be useful to review the discussion of the stretch scale and work scale before using the charts.) When you can do about 75 percent of the exercises in a stage with ease, move on to the next stage, but regularly go back to the exercises you found challenging until you are comfortable with them. If you wish, photocopy the charts to add further weeks to the program.

Good luck! You will be glad you took the opportunity to change your life in a positive way, and I am pleased to have been able to help you do so.

### Basic Routine

| | |
|---|---|
| *Exercise 2-1* | Standing Roll Down |
| *Exercises 3 through 6a* | The Start Stretches |
| *Exercise 9-1* | Hamstring Stretch: Basic |
| *Exercise 12* | Thigh Stretch 2: Standing |
| *Exercise 45* | Spine Stretch |
| *Exercise 50* | Side Leg Lifts |
| *Exercise 16* | Preparation with Cushions |
| *Exercise 18* | The Hundreds: Basic |
| *Exercise 32* | Coordination |
| *Exercise 20* | Single Leg Stretch |
| *Exercise 21* | Double Leg Stretch: Basic |
| *Exercise 25* | The Perfect Abdominal Curl |
| *Exercise 73* | Lumbar Stretch |
| *Exercise 28-2* | Opening Arms |
| *Exercises 29-1, 29-2* | Arm Swings |
| *Exercise 1* | Resting Position (Baby Pose) |

|  | Stage I |
| --- | --- |
| Exercise 2-1 | Standing Roll Down |
| Exercises 3 through 6a | The Start Stretches |
| Exercise 10 | Hamstring Stretch 3 |
| Exercise 13 | Thigh Stretch 3: Kneeling |
| Exercise 45 | Spine Stretch |
| Exercise 44 | Spine Rotation |
| Exercise 48 | The Saw |
| Exercise 16 | Preparation with Cushions |
| Exercise 19-1 | The Hundreds: Intermediate |
| Exercise 25 | The Perfect Abdominal Curl |
| Exercise 76 | Oblique Curls |
| Exercise 20 | Single Leg Stretch |
| Exercise 21 | Double Leg Stretch: Basic |
| Exercise 33 | The Roll-Up |
| Exercise 37 | Rolling Like a Ball |
| Exercise 47-1 | Corkscrew: Basic |
| Exercise 24 | Stomach Stretch |
| Exercises 28-2, 28-3 | Opening Arms / Alternating Arms |
| Exercises 26-1, 26-2 | Ankle Weights |
| Exercises 29-1, 29-2 | Arm Swings |
| Exercise 30 | The Pole |

|  | Stage II |
| --- | --- |
| Exercises 3 through 6a | The Start Stretches |
| Exercise 9-2 | Hamstring Stretch 2 |
| Exercise 13 | Thigh Stretch 3: Kneeling |
| Exercise 76 | Oblique Curls |
| Exercise 23 | Side to Side |
| Exercise 31 | The Hundreds: Alternating Legs |
| Exercise 47-1 | Corkscrew: Basic |
| Exercise 62 | Pendulum |
| Exercise 33 | The Roll-Up |
| Exercise 46 | Open Leg Rocker |
| Exercise 20 | Single Leg Stretch |
| Exercise 36 | Double Leg Stretch 2: Lowering and Raising |
| Exercise 43 | Swimming |
| Exercise 49 | Side Kick 1 |
| Exercise 28-2 through 28-5 | Arm Weights: All Supine Routines |
| Exercises 29-1, 29-2 | Arm Swings |
| Exercise 30 | The Pole |
| Exercise 72 | Stamina Stretch: Advanced |

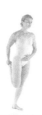

|  | Stage III |  | Stage IV |
|---|---|---|---|
| *Exercises 3 through 6a* | The Start Stretches | *Exercises 3 through 6a* | The Start Stretches |
| *Exercise 9-2* | Hamstring Stretch 2 | *Exercise 9-2* | Hamstring Stretch 2 |
| *Exercise 13* | Thigh Stretch 3: Kneeling | *Exercise 13* | Thigh Stretch 3: Kneeling |
| *Exercise 23* | Side to Side | *Exercise 31* | The Hundreds: Alternating Legs |
| *Exercise 47-2* | Corkscrew 1: Intermediate | *Exercise 25* | The Perfect Abdominal Curl |
| *Exercise 62* | Pendulum | *Exercise 76* | Oblique Curls |
| *Exercise 63* | Neck Curl | *Exercise 63* | Neck Curl |
| *Exercise 76* | Oblique Curls | *Exercise 20* | Single Leg Stretch |
| *Exercise 38* | Crisscross | *Exercise 36* | Double Leg Stretch 2: Lowering and Raising |
| *Exercise 60* | The Hundreds: Lower and Raise | *Exercise 47-3* | Corkscrew 2: Advanced |
| *Exercise 36* | Double Leg Stretch 2: Lowering and Raising | *Exercise 46* | Open Leg Rocker |
| *Exercise 34* | The Roll-Over | *Exercise 34* | The Roll-Over |
| *Exercise 70* | Hip Circles | *Exercise 61* | Roll-Over: Bent Legs |
| *Exercise 65* | Jackknife | *Exercise 53-1* | Teaser 1: Basic |
| *Exercise 58* | Seal | *Exercise 54* | Leg Pull Prone |
| *Exercise 53-1* | Teaser 1: Basic | *Exercise 55* | Leg Pull Supine |
| *Exercise 40* | Single Leg Kick | *Exercise 65* | Jackknife |
| *Exercise 28-2 through 28-5* | Arm Weights: All Supine Routines | *Exercise 59* | Control Balance |
| *Exercises 29-1, 29-2* | Arm Swings | *Exercise 28-2 through 28-5* | Arm Weights: All Supine Routines |
| *Exercise 72* | Stamina Stretch: Advanced | *Exercise 26-1* | Ankle Weights: Outer Thigh (Abductor) |
| *Exercise 30* | The Pole | *Exercises 29-1, 29-2* | Arm Swings |
|  |  | *Exercise 30* | The Pole |
|  |  | *Exercise 72* | Stamina Stretch: Advanced |

## Stage V

| | |
|---|---|
| Exercises 3 through 6a | The Start Stretches |
| Exercise 9-2 | Hamstring Stretch 2 |
| Exercise 13 | Thigh Stretch 3: Kneeling |
| Exercise 60 | The Hundreds: Lower and Raise |
| Exercise 25 | The Perfect Abdominal Curl |
| Exercise 76 | Oblique Curls |
| Exercise 63 | Neck Curl |
| Exercise 36 | Double Leg Stretch 2: Lowering and Raising |
| Exercise 38 | Crisscross |
| Exercise 47-3 | Corkscrew 2: Advanced |
| Exercise 62 | Pendulum |
| Exercise 70 | Hip Circles |
| Exercise 61 | Roll-Over: Bent Legs |
| Exercise 53-2 | Teaser 2 |
| Exercise 54 | Leg Pull Prone |
| Exercise 58 | Seal |
| Exercise 42-2 | Swan Dive 2 |
| Exercise 69-2 | Can-Can Extension |
| Exercise 59 | Control Balance |
| Exercise 66 | Scissors |
| Exercise 74 | Rocking |
| Exercise 49 | Side Kick 1 |
| Exercise 28-2 through 28-5 | Arm Weights: All Supine Routines |
| Exercise 27 | Back of the Thigh: Hamstring/Buttocks |
| Exercises 29-1, 29-2 | Arm Swings |
| Exercise 72 | Stamina Stretch: Advanced |

## Stage VI

| | |
|---|---|
| Exercises 3 through 6a | The Start Stretches |
| Exercise 8-2 | Alternating Calf Stretches |
| Exercise 10 | Hamstring Stretch 3 |
| Exercise 13 | Thigh Stretch 3: Kneeling |
| Exercise 33 | The Roll-Up |
| Exercise 25 | The Perfect Abdominal Curl |
| Exercise 35 | Single Leg Circles |
| Exercise 38 | Crisscross |
| Exercise 36 | Double Leg Stretch 2: (Variation) |
| Exercise 34 | The Roll-Over |
| Exercise 61 | Roll-Over: Bent Legs |
| Exercise 44 | Spine Rotation |
| Exercise 48 | The Saw |
| Exercise 47-3 | Corkscrew 2: Advanced |
| Exercise 42-2 | Swan Dive 2 |
| Exercise 53-3 | Teaser 3 |
| Exercise 66 | Scissors |
| Exercise 67 | Bicycle |
| Exercise 1 | Resting Position (Baby Pose) |
| Exercise 54 | Leg Pull Prone |
| Exercise 55 | Leg Pull Supine |
| Exercise 56 | Side Kick 2 |
| Exercise 57 | Boomerang |
| Exercise 59 | Control Balance |
| Exercise 75-1 | Twist 1 |
| Exercise 28-5 | Arm Circles |
| Exercise 72 | Stamina Stretch: Advanced |
| Exercise 71 | Lying Torso Stretch |
| Exercises 29-1, 29-2 | Arm Swings |
| Exercise 30 | The Pole |

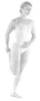

## STUDIO-BASED PILATES PROGRAMS

Beyond the floor routines presented in this book, there are the studio-based Pilates programs. It is always advisable to check to ensure that the studio you wish to attend is a registered, certified studio with an established reputation. Studio-based programs are usually by appointment only. They can give you the full benefit of all of Joe Pilates' work. Under the watchful eye of an instructor, you will be guided through programs suited to your strengths and weaknesses.

Within the studio environment, there are a variety of pieces of equipment with curious names such as the Universal Reformer, the Cadillac, the Wunda Chair, and the Pedi-Pul. The use of specialized equipment challenges your body to advance to a different level. This is not to diminish the importance of the floor routines. As a stand-alone program, the floor routines can be done in any place at any time—a considerable advantage over the equipment-based routines.

## CONCLUSION

When putting Joseph Pilates' techniques to work, you will undoubtedly notice some changes in your body quite soon. To get the most from the program, however, it is also important to be aware of the response your body and muscles are feeding back to you. When you feel you have adequately mastered a specific routine or set of exercises, remain with that program for an additional week to consolidate the connection of the mind and the body on those movements.

Doing this may feel akin to watching a film for the second time and noticing small but important aspects that you were unaware of the first time. If one small aspect of the film were missing, it would not dramatically change the overall message or content of the film. However, if many of these small parts were missing, the film would give the viewer a totally different message! So it is with Pilates work. You, like the viewer of the film, will gradually improve your perception and control over the smaller, once seemingly insignificant, details of the movements. As the parts fuse together to become the whole, your body will regain lost perceptions. Your mind and body will work in unison, and your sense of well-being, both mental and physical, will produce an emotional enthusiasm that your body has not felt for some time—if ever!

I have attempted to be as precise as possible in all the descriptions of the movements. Focus on each of them. As you become more proficient at the exercises, review them after a month, even if you have progressed to the next stage. Scrutinize the descriptions of the exercises to see if you have incorporated every aspect of them into the movement so that your mind and body are getting the full, clear message.

If you apply this level of focus and attention to your practice of the movements, you will not only see the benefits of what Pilates exercises can do for your body; you will become so involved that you will also feel the changes from deep within.

# REFERENCES

Arnheim, Daniel. *Modern Principles of Athletic Training.* St. Louis, MO: Times Mirror, 1989.

Eisen, G., and Freidman, R. *The Pilates Method of Mental and Physical Conditioning.* New York: Warner, 1980 (out of print).

Fitt, S. S. *Dance Kinesiology.* New York: Schirmer Books, 1988.

Howse, J., and Hancock, S. *Dance Technique and Injury Prevention.* London: A & C Black, 1998.

Jordan, Peg, R.N., ed. *Fitness Theory and Practice: The Comprehensive Resource for Fitness Instruction,* 2d ed. Sherman Oaks, CA: Aerobics and Fitness Association of America, 1997.

Kapandji, I. A. *The Physiology of the Joints.* Edinburgh: Churchill Livingston, 1974.

Kendall, F. P., and McCreary, E. K. *Muscles Testing and Function.* Baltimore, MD: Williams & Wilkins, 1993.

Kisner, C., and Colby, L. A. *Therapeutic Exercise.* Philadelphia, PA: F. A. Davis, 1988.

Peterson, L., and Renstrom, P. *Sports Injuries.* Auckland, New Zealand: Methuen, 1988.

Ryan, A. J., and Stephens, R. E. *Dance Medicine.* Chicago: Pluribus Press, 1987.

Winter Griffith, H. *Sports Injuries.* Tucson, AZ: The Body Press, 1986.

*For inquiries on videos, equipment, training,*
*or registering your studio on the Internet, please contact:*

Aussie Pilates and Pilates Institute of Australasia
PO Box 1046
North Sydney NSW 2059
Australia
Phone: +612-8920-2622
Fax: +612-8920-2633
E-mail: info@pilates.net or allan@pilates.net
Website: www.pilates.net

# BASIC ROUTINE EXERCISE CHART

| EXERCISE | WEEK 1 | | | WEEK 2 | | | WEEK 3 | | | WEEK 4 | | | WEEK 5 | | | WEEK 6 | | | WEEK 7 | | |
|---|---|---|---|---|---|---|---|---|---|---|---|---|---|---|---|---|---|---|---|---|---|
| PROGRAM DATE:    /    / | M | W | F | M | W | F | M | W | F | M | W | F | M | W | F | M | W | F | M | W | F |
| #2-2 Standing Roll Down | | | | | | | | | | | | | | | | | | | | | |
| #3 to 6a The Start Stretches | | | | | | | | | | | | | | | | | | | | | |
| #9-1 Hamstring Stretch: Basic | | | | | | | | | | | | | | | | | | | | | |
| #12 Thigh Stretch 2: Standing | | | | | | | | | | | | | | | | | | | | | |
| #45 Spine Stretch | | | | | | | | | | | | | | | | | | | | | |
| #50 Side Leg Lifts | | | | | | | | | | | | | | | | | | | | | |
| #16 Preparation with Cushions | | | | | | | | | | | | | | | | | | | | | |
| #18 The Hundreds: Basic | | | | | | | | | | | | | | | | | | | | | |
| #32 Coordination | | | | | | | | | | | | | | | | | | | | | |
| #20 Single Leg Stretch | | | | | | | | | | | | | | | | | | | | | |
| #21 Double Leg Stretch: Basic | | | | | | | | | | | | | | | | | | | | | |
| #25 The Perfect Abdominal Curl (PAC) | | | | | | | | | | | | | | | | | | | | | |
| #73 Lumbar Stretch | | | | | | | | | | | | | | | | | | | | | |
| #28-2 Opening Arms | | | | | | | | | | | | | | | | | | | | | |
| #29-1, 29-2 Arm Swings | | | | | | | | | | | | | | | | | | | | | |
| #1 Resting Position (Baby Pose) | | | | | | | | | | | | | | | | | | | | | |

# STAGE I EXERCISE CHART

| EXERCISE | WEEK 1 | | | WEEK 2 | | | WEEK 3 | | | WEEK 4 | | | WEEK 5 | | | WEEK 6 | | | WEEK 7 | | |
|---|---|---|---|---|---|---|---|---|---|---|---|---|---|---|---|---|---|---|---|---|---|
| **PROGRAM DATE:  /  /** | M | W | F | M | W | F | M | W | F | M | W | F | M | W | F | M | W | F | M | W | F |
| #2-1 Standing Roll Down | | | | | | | | | | | | | | | | | | | | | |
| #3 through 6a The Start Stretches | | | | | | | | | | | | | | | | | | | | | |
| #10 Hamstring Stretch 3 | | | | | | | | | | | | | | | | | | | | | |
| #13 Thigh Stretch 3: Kneeling | | | | | | | | | | | | | | | | | | | | | |
| #45 Spine Stretch | | | | | | | | | | | | | | | | | | | | | |
| #44 Spine Rotation | | | | | | | | | | | | | | | | | | | | | |
| #48 The Saw | | | | | | | | | | | | | | | | | | | | | |
| #16 Preparation with Cushions | | | | | | | | | | | | | | | | | | | | | |
| #19-1 The Hundreds: Intermediate | | | | | | | | | | | | | | | | | | | | | |
| #25 The Perfect Abdominal Curl (PAC) | | | | | | | | | | | | | | | | | | | | | |
| #76 Oblique Curls | | | | | | | | | | | | | | | | | | | | | |
| #20 Single Leg Stretch | | | | | | | | | | | | | | | | | | | | | |
| #21 Double Leg Stretch: Basic | | | | | | | | | | | | | | | | | | | | | |
| #33 The Roll-Up | | | | | | | | | | | | | | | | | | | | | |
| #37 Rolling Like a Ball | | | | | | | | | | | | | | | | | | | | | |
| #47-1 Corkscrew: Basic | | | | | | | | | | | | | | | | | | | | | |
| #24 Stomach Stretch | | | | | | | | | | | | | | | | | | | | | |
| #28-2, 28-3 Opening Arms, Alternating Arms | | | | | | | | | | | | | | | | | | | | | |
| #26-1, 26-2 Ankle Weights | | | | | | | | | | | | | | | | | | | | | |
| #29-1, 29-2 Arm Swings | | | | | | | | | | | | | | | | | | | | | |
| #30 The Pole | | | | | | | | | | | | | | | | | | | | | |
| | | | | | | | | | | | | | | | | | | | | | |
| | | | | | | | | | | | | | | | | | | | | | |
| | | | | | | | | | | | | | | | | | | | | | |
| | | | | | | | | | | | | | | | | | | | | | |

# STAGE II EXERCISE CHART

| EXERCISE | WEEK 1 | | | WEEK 2 | | | WEEK 3 | | | WEEK 4 | | | WEEK 5 | | | WEEK 6 | | | WEEK 7 | | |
|---|---|---|---|---|---|---|---|---|---|---|---|---|---|---|---|---|---|---|---|---|---|
| PROGRAM DATE:      /      / | M | W | F | M | W | F | M | W | F | M | W | F | M | W | F | M | W | F | M | W | F |
| #3 through 6a The Start Stretches | | | | | | | | | | | | | | | | | | | | | |
| #9-2 Hamstring Stretch 2 | | | | | | | | | | | | | | | | | | | | | |
| #13 Thigh Stretch 3: Kneeling | | | | | | | | | | | | | | | | | | | | | |
| #76 Oblique Curls | | | | | | | | | | | | | | | | | | | | | |
| #23 Side to Side | | | | | | | | | | | | | | | | | | | | | |
| #31 The Hundreds: Alternating Legs | | | | | | | | | | | | | | | | | | | | | |
| #47-1 Corkscrew: Basic | | | | | | | | | | | | | | | | | | | | | |
| #62 Pendulum | | | | | | | | | | | | | | | | | | | | | |
| #33 The Roll-Up | | | | | | | | | | | | | | | | | | | | | |
| #46 Open Leg Rocker | | | | | | | | | | | | | | | | | | | | | |
| #20 Single Leg Stretch | | | | | | | | | | | | | | | | | | | | | |
| #36 Double Leg Stretch 2 | | | | | | | | | | | | | | | | | | | | | |
| #43 Swimming | | | | | | | | | | | | | | | | | | | | | |
| #49 Side Kick 1 | | | | | | | | | | | | | | | | | | | | | |
| #28-2 through 28-5 Arm Weights | | | | | | | | | | | | | | | | | | | | | |
| #29-1, 29-2 Arm Swings | | | | | | | | | | | | | | | | | | | | | |
| #30 The Pole | | | | | | | | | | | | | | | | | | | | | |
| #72 Stamina Stretch: Advanced | | | | | | | | | | | | | | | | | | | | | |
| | | | | | | | | | | | | | | | | | | | | | |
| | | | | | | | | | | | | | | | | | | | | | |
| | | | | | | | | | | | | | | | | | | | | | |

# STAGE III EXERCISE CHART

| EXERCISE | WEEK 1 | | | WEEK 2 | | | WEEK 3 | | | WEEK 4 | | | WEEK 5 | | | WEEK 6 | | | WEEK 7 | | |
|---|---|---|---|---|---|---|---|---|---|---|---|---|---|---|---|---|---|---|---|---|---|
| PROGRAM DATE:      /      / | M | W | F | M | W | F | M | W | F | M | W | F | M | W | F | M | W | F | M | W | F |
| #3 through 6a The Start Stretches | | | | | | | | | | | | | | | | | | | | | |
| #9-2 Hamstring Stretch 2 | | | | | | | | | | | | | | | | | | | | | |
| #13 Thigh Stretch 3: Kneeling | | | | | | | | | | | | | | | | | | | | | |
| #23 Side to Side | | | | | | | | | | | | | | | | | | | | | |
| #47-2 Corkscrew I: Intermediate | | | | | | | | | | | | | | | | | | | | | |
| #62 Pendulum | | | | | | | | | | | | | | | | | | | | | |
| #63 Neck Curl | | | | | | | | | | | | | | | | | | | | | |
| #76 Oblique Curls | | | | | | | | | | | | | | | | | | | | | |
| #38 Crisscross | | | | | | | | | | | | | | | | | | | | | |
| #60 The Hundreds: Lower and Raise | | | | | | | | | | | | | | | | | | | | | |
| #36 Double Leg Stretch 2 | | | | | | | | | | | | | | | | | | | | | |
| #34 The Roll Over | | | | | | | | | | | | | | | | | | | | | |
| #70 Hip Circles | | | | | | | | | | | | | | | | | | | | | |
| #65 Jackknife | | | | | | | | | | | | | | | | | | | | | |
| #58 Seal | | | | | | | | | | | | | | | | | | | | | |
| #53-1 Teaser I: Basic | | | | | | | | | | | | | | | | | | | | | |
| #40 Single Leg Kick | | | | | | | | | | | | | | | | | | | | | |
| #28-2 through 28-5 Arm Weights | | | | | | | | | | | | | | | | | | | | | |
| #29-1, 29-2 Arm Swings | | | | | | | | | | | | | | | | | | | | | |
| #72 Stamina Stretch: Advanced | | | | | | | | | | | | | | | | | | | | | |
| #30 The Pole | | | | | | | | | | | | | | | | | | | | | |
| | | | | | | | | | | | | | | | | | | | | | |
| | | | | | | | | | | | | | | | | | | | | | |
| | | | | | | | | | | | | | | | | | | | | | |
| | | | | | | | | | | | | | | | | | | | | | |

# STAGE IV EXERCISE CHART

| EXERCISE | WEEK 1 | | | WEEK 2 | | | WEEK 3 | | | WEEK 4 | | | WEEK 5 | | | WEEK 6 | | | WEEK 7 | | |
|---|---|---|---|---|---|---|---|---|---|---|---|---|---|---|---|---|---|---|---|---|---|
| PROGRAM DATE:    /    / | M | W | F | M | W | F | M | W | F | M | W | F | M | W | F | M | W | F | M | W | F |
| #3 through 6a The Start Stretches | | | | | | | | | | | | | | | | | | | | | |
| #9-2 Hamstring Stretch 2 | | | | | | | | | | | | | | | | | | | | | |
| #13 Thigh Stretch 3: Kneeling | | | | | | | | | | | | | | | | | | | | | |
| #31 The Hundreds: Alternating Legs | | | | | | | | | | | | | | | | | | | | | |
| #25 The Perfect Abdominal Curl (PAC) | | | | | | | | | | | | | | | | | | | | | |
| #76 Oblique Curls | | | | | | | | | | | | | | | | | | | | | |
| #63 Neck Curl | | | | | | | | | | | | | | | | | | | | | |
| #20 Single Leg Stretch | | | | | | | | | | | | | | | | | | | | | |
| #36 Double Leg Stretch 2 | | | | | | | | | | | | | | | | | | | | | |
| #47-3 Corkscrew 2: Advanced | | | | | | | | | | | | | | | | | | | | | |
| #46 Open Leg Rocker | | | | | | | | | | | | | | | | | | | | | |
| #34 The Roll-Over | | | | | | | | | | | | | | | | | | | | | |
| #61 Roll-Over: Bent Legs | | | | | | | | | | | | | | | | | | | | | |
| #53-1 Teaser I: Basic | | | | | | | | | | | | | | | | | | | | | |
| #54 Leg Pull Prone | | | | | | | | | | | | | | | | | | | | | |
| #55 Leg Pull Supine | | | | | | | | | | | | | | | | | | | | | |
| #65 Jackknife | | | | | | | | | | | | | | | | | | | | | |
| #59 Control Balance | | | | | | | | | | | | | | | | | | | | | |
| #28-2 through 28-5 Arm Weights | | | | | | | | | | | | | | | | | | | | | |
| #26-1 Ankle Weights: Outer Thigh | | | | | | | | | | | | | | | | | | | | | |
| #29-1, 29-2 Arm Swings | | | | | | | | | | | | | | | | | | | | | |
| #30 The Pole | | | | | | | | | | | | | | | | | | | | | |
| #72 Stamina Stretch: Advanced | | | | | | | | | | | | | | | | | | | | | |
| | | | | | | | | | | | | | | | | | | | | | |
| | | | | | | | | | | | | | | | | | | | | | |
| | | | | | | | | | | | | | | | | | | | | | |

# STAGE V EXERCISE CHART

| EXERCISE | WEEK 1 | | | WEEK 2 | | | WEEK 3 | | | WEEK 4 | | | WEEK 5 | | | WEEK 6 | | | WEEK 7 | | |
|---|---|---|---|---|---|---|---|---|---|---|---|---|---|---|---|---|---|---|---|---|---|
| PROGRAM DATE:        /        / | M | W | F | M | W | F | M | W | F | M | W | F | M | W | F | M | W | F | M | W | F |
| #3 through 6a The Start Stretches | | | | | | | | | | | | | | | | | | | | | |
| #9-2 Hamstring Stretch 2 | | | | | | | | | | | | | | | | | | | | | |
| #13 Thigh Stretch 3: Kneeling | | | | | | | | | | | | | | | | | | | | | |
| #60 The Hundreds: Lower and Raise | | | | | | | | | | | | | | | | | | | | | |
| #25 The Perfect Abdominal Curl (PAC) | | | | | | | | | | | | | | | | | | | | | |
| #76 Oblique Curls | | | | | | | | | | | | | | | | | | | | | |
| #63 Neck Curl | | | | | | | | | | | | | | | | | | | | | |
| #36 Double Leg Stretch 2 | | | | | | | | | | | | | | | | | | | | | |
| #38 Crisscross | | | | | | | | | | | | | | | | | | | | | |
| #47-3 Corkscrew 2: Advanced | | | | | | | | | | | | | | | | | | | | | |
| #62 Pendulum | | | | | | | | | | | | | | | | | | | | | |
| #70 Hip Circles | | | | | | | | | | | | | | | | | | | | | |
| #61 Roll-Over: Bent Legs | | | | | | | | | | | | | | | | | | | | | |
| #53-2 Teaser 2 | | | | | | | | | | | | | | | | | | | | | |
| #54 Leg Pull Prone | | | | | | | | | | | | | | | | | | | | | |
| #58 Seal | | | | | | | | | | | | | | | | | | | | | |
| #42-2 Swan Dive 2 | | | | | | | | | | | | | | | | | | | | | |
| #69-2 Can-Can Extension | | | | | | | | | | | | | | | | | | | | | |
| #59 Control Balance | | | | | | | | | | | | | | | | | | | | | |
| #66 Scissors | | | | | | | | | | | | | | | | | | | | | |
| #74 Rocking | | | | | | | | | | | | | | | | | | | | | |
| #49 Side Kick I | | | | | | | | | | | | | | | | | | | | | |
| #28-2 through 28-5 Arm Weights | | | | | | | | | | | | | | | | | | | | | |
| #27 Back of the Thigh | | | | | | | | | | | | | | | | | | | | | |
| #29-I, 29-2 Arm Swings | | | | | | | | | | | | | | | | | | | | | |
| #72 Stamina Stretch: Advanced | | | | | | | | | | | | | | | | | | | | | |
| | | | | | | | | | | | | | | | | | | | | | |
| | | | | | | | | | | | | | | | | | | | | | |
| | | | | | | | | | | | | | | | | | | | | | |

# STAGE VI EXERCISE CHART

| EXERCISE | WEEK 1 | | | WEEK 2 | | | WEEK 3 | | | WEEK 4 | | | WEEK 5 | | | WEEK 6 | | | WEEK 7 | | |
|---|---|---|---|---|---|---|---|---|---|---|---|---|---|---|---|---|---|---|---|---|---|
| PROGRAM DATE:    /    / | M | W | F | M | W | F | M | W | F | M | W | F | M | W | F | M | W | F | M | W | F |
| #3 through 6a The Start Stretches | | | | | | | | | | | | | | | | | | | | | |
| #8-2 Alternating Calf Stretches | | | | | | | | | | | | | | | | | | | | | |
| #10 Hamstrings Stretch 3 | | | | | | | | | | | | | | | | | | | | | |
| #13 Thigh Stretch 3: Kneeling | | | | | | | | | | | | | | | | | | | | | |
| #33 The Roll-Up | | | | | | | | | | | | | | | | | | | | | |
| #25 The Perfect Abdominal Curl (PAC) | | | | | | | | | | | | | | | | | | | | | |
| #35 Single Leg Circles | | | | | | | | | | | | | | | | | | | | | |
| #38 Crisscross | | | | | | | | | | | | | | | | | | | | | |
| #36 Double Leg Stretch 2 (Variation) | | | | | | | | | | | | | | | | | | | | | |
| #34 The Roll Over | | | | | | | | | | | | | | | | | | | | | |
| #61 Roll Over: Bent Legs | | | | | | | | | | | | | | | | | | | | | |
| #44 Spine Rotation | | | | | | | | | | | | | | | | | | | | | |
| #48 The Saw | | | | | | | | | | | | | | | | | | | | | |
| #47-3 Corkscrew 2: Advanced | | | | | | | | | | | | | | | | | | | | | |
| #42-2 Swan Dive 2 | | | | | | | | | | | | | | | | | | | | | |
| #53-3 Teaser 3 | | | | | | | | | | | | | | | | | | | | | |
| #66 Scissors | | | | | | | | | | | | | | | | | | | | | |
| #67 Bicycle | | | | | | | | | | | | | | | | | | | | | |
| #1 Resting Position (Baby Pose) | | | | | | | | | | | | | | | | | | | | | |
| #54 Leg Pull Prone | | | | | | | | | | | | | | | | | | | | | |
| #55 Leg Pull Supine | | | | | | | | | | | | | | | | | | | | | |
| #56 Side Kick 2 | | | | | | | | | | | | | | | | | | | | | |
| #57 Boomerang | | | | | | | | | | | | | | | | | | | | | |
| #59 Control Balance | | | | | | | | | | | | | | | | | | | | | |
| #75-1 Twist 1 | | | | | | | | | | | | | | | | | | | | | |
| #28-5 Arm Circles | | | | | | | | | | | | | | | | | | | | | |
| #72 Stamina Stretch: Advanced | | | | | | | | | | | | | | | | | | | | | |
| #71 Lying Torso Stretch | | | | | | | | | | | | | | | | | | | | | |
| #29-1, 29-2 Arm Swings | | | | | | | | | | | | | | | | | | | | | |
| #30 The Pole | | | | | | | | | | | | | | | | | | | | | |

# EXERCISE CHART

| EXERCISE | WEEK 1 | | | WEEK 2 | | | WEEK 3 | | | WEEK 4 | | | WEEK 5 | | | WEEK 6 | | | WEEK 7 | | |
|---|---|---|---|---|---|---|---|---|---|---|---|---|---|---|---|---|---|---|---|---|---|
| PROGRAM DATE:    /    / | M | W | F | M | W | F | M | W | F | M | W | F | M | W | F | M | W | F | M | W | F |
| | | | | | | | | | | | | | | | | | | | | | |
| | | | | | | | | | | | | | | | | | | | | | |
| | | | | | | | | | | | | | | | | | | | | | |
| | | | | | | | | | | | | | | | | | | | | | |
| | | | | | | | | | | | | | | | | | | | | | |
| | | | | | | | | | | | | | | | | | | | | | |
| | | | | | | | | | | | | | | | | | | | | | |
| | | | | | | | | | | | | | | | | | | | | | |
| | | | | | | | | | | | | | | | | | | | | | |
| | | | | | | | | | | | | | | | | | | | | | |
| | | | | | | | | | | | | | | | | | | | | | |
| | | | | | | | | | | | | | | | | | | | | | |

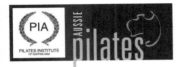

# Learn Pilates in the comfort of your own home!

All prices and shipping charges for this page are in Australian dollars.
Send all orders for these products to PIA at the address below.

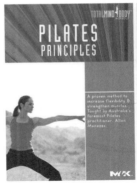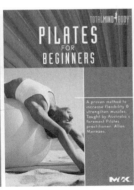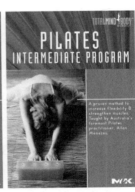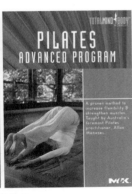

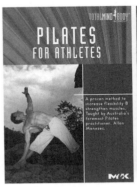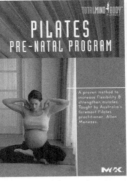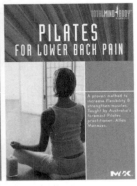

*All prices and shipping charges for this page are in Australian dollars. Send all orders and payments for these products to PIA at the address below.*

**Order Online!**
In North America visit:
www.m-2k.com
For all other areas visit:
www.pilates.net

**For International shipping charges see www.pilates.net. Order online for more special offers.**

- - - - - - - - - - - - - - - - - - - - - - - - - - - - - - - - - -

Name: _____

Adress: _____

Zip Code: _____ State: _____ Country: _____

Telephone: _____ Fax: _____ E-Mail: _____

*Please Send Me:*

☐ 1. **Pilates Principles**: $32.95 + S&H          ☐ 2. **Pilates Intermediate Program**: $32.95 + S&H

☐ 3. **Pilates for Beginners**: $32.95 + S&H          ☐ 4. **Pilates Advanced Program**: $32.95 + S&H

☐ **The Complete Pilates Workout:** *(4 DVD set includes Principles, Beginners, Intermediate & Advanced)*: $99.95 + S&H

☐ **Pilates for Lower Back Pain**: $39.95 + S&H

☐ **Pilates Pre-Natal Program**: $39.95 + S&H

☐ **Pilates for Athletes**: $39.95 + S&H

Payment Details: *(Only credit card payments are accepted with this order form.)*

☐ Shipping: $ _____

☐ Credit Card Amount: $ _____  ☐ Visa  ☐ Mastercard

Card # _____ Expiration Date: _____

Name on Card: _____ Signature on Card: _____

Send completed form to: Pilates Institute of Australasia (PIA), PO Box 1046, North Sydney NSW 2059, Australia or Fax: +612 8920-2633.
If you have any queries, call the Pilates Institute of Australasia at Tel: +612 8920-2622; email: info@pilates.net or purchase online from: www.pilates.net

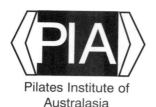

**Pilates Institute of Australasia**

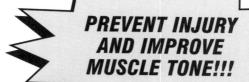

**PREVENT INJURY AND IMPROVE MUSCLE TONE!!!**

# ISOTONER™

The Isotoner™ is the ideal affordable "gym in a bag" that can help you increase your:

- *Arms and upper body*
- *Leg line*
- *Suppleness*
- *Strength*

*Priced at just $29.95*

The Isotoner™ is the ideal resistance aid for basic, intermediate and advanced Pilates floor routine exercises. The Isotoner™ is compact, affordable and easy to use.

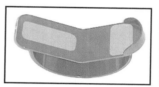

# STRETCHIT!

StretchIt! is for every serious athlete who uses their ankles – that's all of you! Prevent injury and stretch your calves the easiest way with this sturdy product. Made from high grade aluminium, it can take weights of up to 440lbs (200kgs), yet weighs only 2.2lbs (1kg)!

*Priced at just $149*

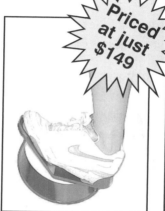

Indestructible under normal use, StretchIt! has a lifetime guarantee.

✂------------------------------------------------------------

Name: _____

Address: _____

State: _____ Zip Code: _____ Country: _____

Telephone: _____ Fax: _____ Email: _____

**Please send me...**

❏ **1 x ISOTONER**™ for $29.95 + $4.50 s&h     ❏ **2 x ISOTONER**™ for $49.95 + $9.00 s&h

**NOTE: Isotoners™ are available in three different resistances—please indicate which:** ⌐ **Light (green)** ⌐ **Medium (blue)** ⌐ **Heavy (silver)**

❏ **1 x STRETCHIT!** for $149 + $33.50 s&h

**Payment details...** (only credit card payments are accepted)

Amount: $_____     ❏ Visa   ❏ MasterCard

Card #: ____ ____ ____ ____ ____ ____ ____ ____ ____ ____ ____ ____ ____ ____ ____ ____     Expiration Date: _____

Name on Card: _____

Signature on Card: _____

Send completed form plus payment to: **Pilates Institute of Australasia (PIA), PO Box 1046, North Sydney NSW 2059, Australia or Fax: (+612) 9267 8226.**
If you have any queries, call the Pilates Institute of Australasia at Tel: (+612) 9267 8223; email: allan@pilates.net, or order online: www.pilates.net

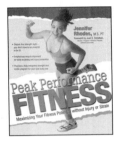
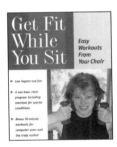
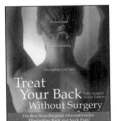
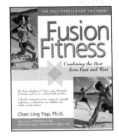
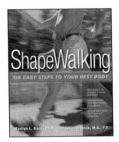
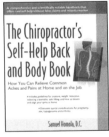

# ORDER FORM

10%    DISCOUNT on orders of $50 or more —
20%    DISCOUNT on orders of $150 or more —
30%    DISCOUNT on orders of $500 or more —
*On cost of books for fully prepaid orders*

NAME

ADDRESS

CITY/STATE                                              ZIP/POSTCODE

PHONE                          COUNTRY (outside of U.S.)

| TITLE | QTY | PRICE | TOTAL |
|---|---|---|---|
| *Joseph H. Pilates' Techniques... (paperback)* | | @  $17.95 | |

*Prices subject to change without notice*

Please list other titles below:

| | | | |
|---|---|---|---|
| | | @  $ | |
| | | @  $ | |
| | | @  $ | |
| | | @  $ | |
| | | @  $ | |
| | | @  $ | |

Please order all Pilates Institute of Australasia products
directly from them, using their order forms.

**Shipping Costs**

*By Priority Mail, first book
$4.50, each additional book
$1.00
By UPS and to Canada, first
book $5.50, each additional
book $1.50
For rush orders and other
countries call us at (510)
865-5282*

TOTAL                          _____
Less discount @_____%      ( _____ )
TOTAL COST OF BOOKS        _____
Calif. residents add sales tax    _____
Shipping & handling        _____
**TOTAL ENCLOSED**         _____

*Please pay in U.S. funds only*

❑ Check  ❑ Money Order  ❑ Visa  ❑ MasterCard  ❑ Discover

Card # _____  Exp. date _____

Signature _____

*Complete and mail to:*
**Hunter House Inc., Publishers**
PO Box 2914, Alameda CA 94501-0914
**Orders: (800) 266-5592   www.hunterhouse.com**
Phone (510) 865-5282 Fax (510) 865-4295
❑ Check here to receive our FREE book catalog

CPM2 5/04